The International Behavioural and Social Sciences Library

DISCUSSIONS ON CHILD
DEVELOPMENT

I0128484

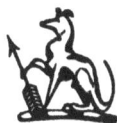

TAVISTOCK

The International Behavioural and Social Sciences Library

CHILD DEVELOPMENT
In 9 Volumes

DISCUSSIONS ON CHILD DEVELOPMENT

Volume Three

EDITED BY J M TANNER
AND BÄRBEL INHELDER

Routledge
Taylor & Francis Group

LONDON AND NEW YORK

First published in 1958 by
Tavistock Publications Limited

Published in 2001 by
Routledge
2 Park Square, Milton Park, Abingdon, Oxfordshire OX14 4RN
711 Third Avenue, New York, NY 10017

First issued in paperback 2014

Routledge is an imprint of the Taylor and Francis Group, an informa business

© 1958 Tavistock Publications Limited

British Library Cataloguing in Publication Data
A CIP catalogue record for this book
is available from the British Library

Discussions on Child Development
ISBN 0-415-26403-0
Child Development: 9 Volumes
ISBN 0-415-26506-1
The International Behavioural and Social Sciences Library
112 Volumes
ISBN 0-415-25670-4

ISBN 13: 978-1-138-87581-4 (pbk)
ISBN 13: 978-0-415-26403-7 (hbk)

DISCUSSIONS ON
Child Development

A Consideration of the Biological, Psychological, and
Cultural Approaches to the Understanding
of Human Development and Behaviour

EDITORS

J. M. TANNER

M.D., D.SC., D.P.M.

Senior Lecturer in Growth and Development
Institute of Child Health, University of London

BÄRBEL INHELDER

Professor of Child Psychology, University of Geneva

VOLUME THREE

The Proceedings of the Third Meeting of the
World Health Organization Study Group
on the Psychobiological Development of the Child
Geneva 1955

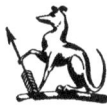

TAVISTOCK PUBLICATIONS LTD.

First published in 1958
by Tavistock Publications Limited
2 Park Square, Milton Park,
Abingdon, Oxon, OX14 4RN

MEMBERS OF STUDY GROUP

DR. A. RÉMOND   *Electrophysiology*

Chargé de Recherches
Centre national de la Recherche
scientifique, Paris

DR. J. M. TANNER   *Human Biology*

Senior Lecturer in Growth and Development
Institute of Child Health
University of London

DR. W. GREY WALTER   *Electrophysiology*

Director of Research
Burden Neurological Institute
Bristol

RENÉ ZAZZO   *Psychology*

Directeur de Laboratoire de
Psychobiologie de l'Enfant
Institut des Hautes Études
Paris

GUESTS

DR. D. BUCKLE   *Psychiatry*
Regional Officer for Mental Health
Regional Office for Europe
World Health Organization
Copenhagen

PROFESSOR ERIK ERIKSON   *Psychoanalysis*
Austen Riggs Center
Stockbridge, Mass.
and
Dept. of Psychiatry
University of Pittsburgh School of Medicine

DR. JULIAN S. HUXLEY   *Biology*
Formerly Director-General, U.N.E.S.C.O.
London

DR. RAYMOND DE SAUSSURE   *Psychoanalysis*
Geneva

PREFACE

Those who have read the first two volumes of this series will already know that the Study Group at its first meeting heard and discussed presentations from representatives of various different scientific disciplines which study some aspect of child development or matters relevant to it, and that at its second meeting the presentations, and the discussions, were focused less specifically on the contributions of different disciplines and more upon aspects of child development in which several disciplines are interested, including such matters as the existence of recognizable stages in development and the phenomenon of learning in immature or developing organisms, and particularly learning under stress.

The third meeting focused upon two related topics: the development of sex differences and the development of individuality or ego identity, and the pattern of psychological development which leads up to it.

The discussion of the first of these topics was based upon two presentations: one by Margaret Mead of comparative data from different societies which might throw light upon the extent to which sex differences were determined by nature or by nurture, and the second by Erik Erikson on sex differences in the play constructions of adolescents.

The opening presentations of the second topic were also made by Erik Erikson. In addition to Mr. Erikson two other distinguished guests joined the Group for this meeting: Dr. Julian Huxley and Dr. Raymond de Saussure.

As on previous occasions the meeting, which was held in Geneva in 1955, provided for its participants a week of stimulating and vigorous discussion which, since it was conducted as usual in both English and French, could not have been possible without simultaneous interpretation equipment and the remarkable ability of the W.H.O. interpreters to follow, and communicate simultaneously in a different language, discussion which, as the reader will find, was often of an exceedingly technical nature and couched in the terminologies of a variety of different scientific disciplines.

To the participant observer it also seemed that a change in the Study Group itself contributed to the success of the meeting. At its first meeting in 1953 its members had comparatively little knowledge of the interests. the methods. and the theoretical models of those in other disciplines who studied the problems of child development; by the third meeting their understanding of each other's work was sufficient to enable them to appreciate and to criticize the formulation of those who worked in other fields and to consider its relevance to their own. For this development in mutual understanding the Group owes much to its Chairman—Dr. Frank Fremont-Smith.

The production of the English transcript of the extensive bilingual discussion depended upon the excellent sound recording facilities provided by W.H.O. and above all on Mrs. J. Moser of the Organization's Mental Health Section whose combination of linguistic ability, technical knowledge, and keen interest in the work of the Group has enabled the contributions of its French-speaking members to be rendered in a sensitive and accurate English translation in these volumes.

Dr. Tanner and Professor Inhelder have edited the transcript of this third meeting and have shown again their ability to reduce a week of discussion to the bounds of a single volume while preserving to a surprising degree its content and its savour.

Leeds University   G. R. HARGREAVES

CONTENTS

The Childhood Genesis of Sex Differences in Behaviour

CANDAU (Director-General, World Health Organization):
This is the third meeting of this research study group. It is to be devoted to consideration of socio-cultural influences affecting psychological development.

I am very glad to welcome once more to Geneva the original members of the Group and also our three distinguished guests: Mr. Erik Erikson of the United States, Dr. Raymond de Saussure of Geneva, and Dr. Julian Huxley of the United Kingdom.

Members who have been present at previous meetings of this Group already know its purpose, but it is worth emphasizing, for the benefit of our guests, that the Group is not intended to make decisions or recommendations on any subject to anyone. Its aim is to increase mutual understanding between eminent exponents of the many different disciplines that study child development and its disorders, particularly in the fields of psychology and physiology.

It only remains necessary for me to wish the Group, under its Chairman, Dr. Frank Fremont-Smith, a stimulating and enjoyable meeting.

FREMONT-SMITH:
We might remind our guests and ourselves that we operate on an extremely informal basis. As Dr. Candau said, the purpose of our meeting is to increase mutual understanding. I think that we should feel rather free to interrupt one another, and your Chairman will only step in occasionally when more than three speak at once. In this way we aim to create a group discussion rather than a series of speeches to which the group gives polite attention.

Now to begin with we would like our three guests to tell us a little bit about themselves. (The regular members of the group introduced

13

themselves in a similar fashion at the first meeting, recorded in Vol. I.) How did they happen to arrive at the kind of interest that led them, on the one hand, to be invited to come here and on the other hand, and even more importantly, to accept?

HUXLEY:

I had better begin with the age of about seven when I found myself fascinated by watching birds which were nesting under the eaves of our house just, I think, because they were alive but had a different kind of life from my own. I think it is fair to say that I have always been interested in the fact of difference and the variety of life and of the world as a whole. It was only later that I got interested in the converse problem of what unity there was to be found in it all, and from about 1934 onwards I spent most of my time trying to make a synthesis of the different approaches to biological evolution. How I got into biology was quite accidental. When I was at school I got to a stage where one could take a certain amount of work in a special subject of choice, and I wrote, I remember, to my parents and said 'wouldn't it be a good thing if I took German', because it was then thought I might go into the Civil Service. They wrote back and said 'no, you can go to Germany later and learn German, why don't you take biology?' Well, the biology master at Eton was a genius, and after two months I knew I was going to be a biologist.

Of course, I wouldn't have been invited to join this Group if I had been a biologist interested solely in subhuman phenomena, but I remember that over 40 years ago, when I was teaching in Texas, I had to give a public lecture, and as I had already begun to think of the problem of continuity and discontinuity in evolution I chose as my subject the critical point between subhuman and human evolution. The first book that I published, before the first World War, was about biological individuality, which I am delighted to hear Konrad Lorenz has been re-reading and even finding interesting still. Then I think I am right in saying that the first occasion on which a displacement activity was scientifically recorded was in my long paper on the courtship of the Great Crested Grebe, published 41 years ago. I didn't know what a displacement activity was, but I recorded the facts of this unexplained phenomenon; and I spent a lot of time during the next 25 years, off and on, working on the biological function of epigamic and throat display in birds and their relation to sexual selection. Meanwhile, I was also interested in the various aspects of experimental embryology and growth, especially relative growth of parts; I found myself driven to put forward the

14

idea that the basis for various aspects of growth and development must be sought in some form of field involving gradients. So I was naturally much interested in the then new ideas of the Gestalt psychologists, who were also thinking in field terms, and were interested in psychological development. Then I found myself dealing with a curious feature of some organisms such as Ascidians and Coelenterates—their peculiar faculty of physical regression or dedifferentiation: they not only get smaller but they regress to a simpler stage if you maltreat them in various ways—and this led me to read up all I could about psychological regression. Later I am afraid I strayed rather outside the biological field: in 1928, I think it was, I rushed into print with a book on religion as a natural phenomenon instead of a supernatural one—Religion without Revelation, I called it. And later on I had wished on me the task of relating ethics to evolution by the Vice-Chancellor of Oxford, who invited me to deliver the Romanes lecture 50 years after my grandfather had given his celebrated one on evolution and ethics, and to treat of the same subject, so I had to do some thinking about that problem. Recently, I have had to do some thinking about an equally difficult problem for a mere biologist—the Wenner-Gren Foundation have asked me to write something on anthropology from the angle of an evolutionary biologist.

Then, the fact of being in Geneva reminds me that in 1925 I attended what was, I believe, the first international conference on population, here in Geneva. Ever since then I have been deeply interested in this problem, which I think is one of the world's most serious problems, psychologically as well as politically and socially.

You asked me, Mr. Chairman, why I was willing to come here. I should think that the answer is pretty obvious. This type of meeting seems to me absolutely essential in the present state of the world. We have got to a state where we can't progress if we each of us stay in our own little specialisms. I am sure we have got to a stage where we must somehow organize the synthesis of different branches of knowledge. People say that science has got too specialized for that. I don't believe this is true. Only you have got to find out the technique of getting representatives of different branches together, of getting mutual understanding, and of organizing the synthesis. When I heard about this group here, I thought, well, this certainly is extraordinarily interesting because here we have ethologists and psychologists, medical men and biologists, physiologists and psychiatrists, all interested in one general problem, and I shall be most interested to see how a group of this sort functions, as well as to hear the results of its deliberations.

15

FREMONT-SMITH:

Now, if I may I will ask Erik Erikson to tell us a little bit about himself.

ERIKSON:

I should state first what I am doing. I am a psychoanalyst who divides his time up about equally between psychoanalytic psychotherapy, the training of young doctors for psychoanalysis, and research. The psychotherapy fuses, of course, with research, for what in most of your fields is experimentation, in our field is the attempt to delineate previously incurable mental states in such a way that they become more curable. I work at a small sanitarium in the Berkshire Hills in New England which is also a research institute. There some of us specialize in work with young 'borderline cases', which means young people on the brink of schizophrenia or psychopathy. Ours is an open hospital which deliberately takes certain chances with the patients in order to understand them not as victims of fatalistic diagnosis, but as individual cases of what I will describe in a later meeting as identity diffusion, i.e., a particular difficulty attending the age of youth, and this particularly where society and family have let young people down in specific ways. In addition to intensive psychotherapy, we experiment by giving the patients a responsible voice in the management of the 'hospital environment', and by developing individual ways of work productivity. This is my wife's domain. I am also a visiting professor in the Medical School in Pittsburgh where I learn about patients with similar symptoms but different social backgrounds.

I should have said at the beginning that I do not speak English, but a form of American. This may make it difficult for you to understand what I say, yet it is intrinsically related to our general subject. For my friends (my very best friends) will tell you that I am the best case illustration of an identity diffusion, that is of the clinical picture which I will describe to you when my time comes. Identify diffusion results from the inability to integrate one's childhood identifications and adolescent tasks. Well, I was born a Dane. But my father died around the time of my birth, and my mother and I seem to have travelled a lot. When I was three years old I fell ill in a city in Southern Germany. We stayed there, because my mother married my paediatrician. This, I think, has been a most decisive event as regards my later identity development.

FREMONT-SMITH:

Was it a psychosomatic illness?

16

ERIKSON:

Well, I certainly needed a father. Later, my stepfather very much wanted me to be a doctor. But I decided to become an artist.

The secret identification with the paediatrician appeared only in the fact that I specialized in baby pictures and portraits of children. To do such portraits, I went to Vienna and joined a friend as a tutor in an American family which was close to Freud. Eventually, I was trained as a child analyst under Anna Freud and August Aichhorn and graduated as a psychoanalyst from the Vienna Institute. In Vienna, I also married an American woman of Canadian origin, and we moved to Cambridge, Massachusetts. One of our neighbours was Frank Fremont-Smith through whose interest I received my first medical school and hospital appointments. From then on I have been living in the medical world as much as anybody could who is not a medical man and my stepfather, the paediatrician, was as right as anybody could be who was wrong! And you may well see that I had to make out of identity diffusion a virtue—and a subject.

Now, as for my preoccupations, the daily work of a psychoanalyst is in many ways cut out for him. But I would mention that the artist in me keeps paying special attention to the 'configurational level', by which I mean something which in psychoanalysis is between the obvious, manifest behaviour and the latent, hidden meaning. I will present examples of children's play, trying to show what a child is saying by the way in which it behaves in space, and how it arranges toys and dolls. In work with very small children, it helps tremendously if one is not restricted to listening but if one can observe, and I think it was here that my paediatric and artistic sides came to some kind of agreement. This was further enhanced when I met Margaret Mead and a few other anthropologists and found that in comparing configurations we spoke, as it were, a similar language and could speak about childhood and culture patterns in a way that eventually made dynamic sense also. Thus I became interested in the relationship of human motivation as discovered by psychoanalysis to people's world images and economic systems: what people are hunting and where and how. Having studied two American Indian tribes, it seemed only right to study American children who were neither Indians nor patients. So I participated for a number of years in a longitudinal study of Californian children to try to understand their particular development in that rapidly growing area which was rather freshly settled compared to the rest of the world.

My special interest is this. In psychoanalysis, which originated in the era of enlightenment and individualism, the original emphasis

B 17

was on the dichotomy between the individual and his society, almost in the sense that environment as such was essentially hostile to the individual. This, of course, was an ideological distortion of what Freud, at given stages of his studies, had pointed out. Today, the analysis of the ego makes it very clear that no individual could possibly exist, or grow strong, or, indeed, become an individual without society. But how does he do it, and how does society keep the bargain? I think that the psychoanalysis of the ego permits a new approach to the contract between individual and society. If I may make in conclusion what I hope to be a challenging statement, I think I came here with the expectation of learning from this particular group a new approach to the ethological nature of love. But by this I do not mean only the mutuality between mother and child, and not only the pact of personal love, but also such psychosocial contracts as forms of truth, styles of honesty, kinds of justice. All of these seem as indispensable for the human child's development as the life-preserving features of the physical environment.

FREMONT-SMITH:

If I may I will now call upon Dr. Raymond de Saussure to tell us about himself—it is a great joy to see an old friend from New York who was over from Geneva and is now back here in Geneva with us.

DE SAUSSURE:

Unfortunately, although I am a psychiatrist and a psychoanalyst, I am not able to bring you an account of such a miraculous or spectacular cure as that which Mr. Erikson underwent at the age of three years—his own cure and the cure of his mother were certainly determining factors in his career. So I will stay within more modest limits, and as we have been asked to give a biography which begins with the early years I shall keep to the classical pattern of psychoanalysis—although Dr. Hargreaves asked us not to be too classical —and I will tell you here of my oral stage, my anal stage and my genital stage.

In my oral stage I was very greedy and I think I was able to sublimate a part of this greediness in the desire to read and study later on. The anal stage was characterized for me by a liking for collecting and studying butterflies, and throughout my adolescence (which is a rather late anal stage) I developed this liking for making collections. The genital stage was very much retarded too, this time through Calvinism and its very strong influences to which I was subjected, so that I had to go off to Vienna to be analysed by Freud and to get

18

rid of some of these overpowering ancestral influences. I was very grateful to him, but I did not immediately realize the full value of this method and returned later to Berlin to undergo a second analysis with Dr. Alexander and to follow courses at the institute.

Actually, I owe my interest in psychoanalysis to Théodore Flournoy who was Professor of Psychology here in Geneva. Immediately after my secondary schooling I became deeply interested in his lectures in which, as early as 1914, he used to expound his psychoanalytic theories. My interest turned very quickly first towards the similarities or the concordances which could exist between the ideas of Freud and Jean Piaget. Here there were two points of view about psychology, two genetic points of view, which seemed to complement each other but which unfortunately had previously been put in opposition to each other. During meetings of French-speaking psychoanalysts I had the opportunity of establishing the first connexions, which later on were well worked out by my friend Charles Odier. Another of my interests was to find the possible relationships between certain social structures and certain forms of neuroses (de Saussure, 1929, 1946).

In my book on the Greek Miracle (de Saussure, 1939) I tried to show why scientific civilization was born in Greece rather than elsewhere. My great interest for all the problems of psychology intermingled with those of biology and politics dates from this time. When I went to the United States in 1940 I had the very great privilege of following many inter-disciplinary discussions where psychological, biological, social and political points of view were intermixed.

For this reason I was extremely happy to receive your invitation which corresponds to one of my major interests. I am looking forward immensely to hearing you and I shall try to contribute in my modest degree to your discussions.

FREMONT-SMITH:

Now we have had our introductions, and begun to group, if one can use that word in the intransitive sense. May I turn to you, Margaret, to open the discussion and do it in your own way—you have quite a period of time, two-and-a-half days. The principle, as you know, is to ask the opener to have each day about 20 minutes of material to present and then if they are really successful in the two-and-a-half days they can't get it all presented because of the discussion which is stirred up.

MEAD:

My task now is to describe what light anthropology can shed on
19

the occurrence of what can be regarded as universal sex differences, however differently these may be patterned and institutionalized in different societies. Conversely, I want to provide a way of removing from our present formulation the culturally limited ethnocentric and provincial material on sex differences. This means that I will use for the most part extreme anthropological cases. If I talk about something that is reasonably widespread and universal it would be impossible for me to give you any detail—for example of the fact that mothers breast-feed babies in all parts of the world. So I shall select the most interesting cases, with your understanding that these are extreme and that we assume, in between, the existence of a very large number of less peculiar, less extreme behaviour patterns.

I think that we should really start with the child's realization of the fact that it is a human being, which is, I think, more important than its realization of which sex it is. For instance, in Bali, people are unwilling to treat a child under three months as a human being; the new-born baby has no name, is not allowed to enter a temple and is called a rat or a caterpillar. Then there are societies that identify children with vegetables or with animals for a very long time and undoubtedly change the individual's sense of who they are and what it means to be a human being.

Coming to sex differences, I think that we will find it useful to consider first those differences between the sexes which have occurred in every society to date, but which may nevertheless be modifiable. Until recently, for instance, human infants have been breast-fed, the feeding bottle being a comparatively recent invention. As long as human infants had to be breast-fed by human mothers there was a universal condition of the early differentiation of sex roles, as children of both sexes were fed by a creature of one sex everywhere. This ceased to be universal as soon as the feeding-bottle was invented. What looked like a very long and very important element in the differentiation of the two sexes could be wiped out by a single invention. Equally, of course, it could be restored. Thus all of the points that are connected with maternal care of children, or care by another female such as a nurse, a wet-nurse, a foster mother, etc., although they have been almost universal to date, may nevertheless be a biological condition which society is able to abrogate, or change. The whole question of social inventions which may alter present differentiation of the sexes is exceedingly important.

On the other hand, a great proportion of our present psychological theory about differences between the sexes is based upon the presence of clothing. Psychoanalytic theories that are based on the importance of the revelation of the anatomy of adults, or of your little brother, if you are a little girl, of course are based on the experience of the child in a clothed society where the child encounters only the bodies of small children and the bodies of parents in most cases, with the intervening link left out. In any society where the people don't wear clothes, the situation is very different. The little boy may be alarmed by the contrast between the size of his own and his father's genitals but certainly not in the same way as in clothed society because he sees every possible other size in between and is continually assured that, if he continues to grow, he will eventually get larger. In the same way the presence of pregnancy is conspicuous, and in a primitive society where there are no large buildings and no other achievements, pregnancy is one of the most conspicuous events in the life of the child. We have to bear in mind all the time the extent to which our theory of sex differences is limited by conditions in our own society at present.

I want also to stress that, because the early upbringing of girls and boys by one or both sexes is a major device by which the child's sense of its sex identity is carried, every aspect of sex differences in the life of the society (including the after-life) becomes important in the sex differentiation of the growing boy and girl. For instance, you may live in a society where women have no soul, or you may live in a society where women are only permitted into heaven by way of their husband's soul, as with the folk belief in eastern European Jewry that if a man was a good man and the woman had been a good wife she could go to heaven with him and was permitted to sit at his feet for ever and listen to him talk. This image of heaven is bound to affect very small girls in many ways, as their mothers either look forward with pleasure to this picture or possibly chafe against it. Or consider the Aztec belief that a specially honoured place was reserved in the next world for those men who died in battle and women who died in childbirth; the blood of the slain was equated—men or women. The influence such a picture must have on a small girl or a small boy must be quite different from that of a village where childbirth, menstrual huts, latrines and pigs are put over the edge of the village in a rough, rainy, muddy, precipitous spot, and the place is called the 'evil place'. The social structure will affect children from the very start. In some Mohammedan countries, for instance, the only tie the mother has to the child is the milk-tie. If she breast-feeds the child, that gives her a right to it. The fact that she gave it house room in the foetal stage is regarded as irrelevant; the child is the father's child and the mother runs a boarding house. This affects the whole structure—what happens in divorce, the father's rights to the child, and so forth.

When we consider how a girl learns that she is a girl, and a boy learns that he is a boy, we must remember that a whole series of attitudes are prefigured for them. In the way they are treated, the way they are named, whether the family are glad a boy is born or whether they say, 'when a girl is born everyone weeps and ruin is brought on the house.' From what we know about the relationship of a mother's attitude during lactation, we may expect that a girl who is born as a ruin in the house probably imbibes feelings about ruin during this stage of lactation. Similarly, we must consider even the prenatal period. If a mother knows, from the moment that she is pregnant, that if her child is a girl its chances of life are very different from its chances of life as a boy, this becomes an important psychological distinction; important to the degree that there are psychosomatic connections between the expectation of the mother and the well-being or degree of activity of the foetus. Even the last moment of birth, just before you know whether the child is a girl or a boy, is an exceedingly tense moment for the whole group of women gathered around who know that when they say 'it's a girl', the father will probably say 'abandon it', or 'kill it'. This creates all through pregnancy an attitude in the mother of two kinds of expectancy, which then may culminate one way or the other at birth.

BOWLBY:
May I interrupt? All the instances that you have given us have been adverse to females; are there similar illustrations adverse to males?

MEAD:
There are the societies that expect the male to die earlier. This was characteristic of the Plains Indians of North America—the Cheyennes, for instance. The boy was indulged because he was going to die. Now, if the indulgence for the boy child is phrased that he was superior or stronger that is one thing, but if it is phrased as 'we give you the special titbits from the table because you are going to die' that is another. It is quite possible we might arrive at the same position in the United States at present, for it has been very widely advertised that male expectation of life is something like five years less than the female, and that all women are going to be widows with large bank accounts while their husbands are dead. I should think that a small boy who is brought up in a household with seven widows with large bank accounts and also read this continually in the press, would begin to get a picture of the male sex as deprived. Or in a period when there is a military draft, affecting males and not

22

females or affecting them very differentially, there may again be a sense of the male being condemned to a more dangerous, a more hazardous or a shorter life.

BOWLBY:
It would be necessary to distinguish, then, between misfortunes connected with the one sex and social devaluation of that sex.

MEAD:
Yes, I think one should. But in using the word 'misfortune' you, yourself, were reflecting our point of view that people don't get killed in war except unluckily. This is the European position—that people come back from war unless they are unfortunate enough to be killed. But there are many cultures in which you don't come back from war unless you are peculiarly lucky and so don't get killed—Japan, for instance; the assumption in Japan is that when you go into the Army you are dead; if you happen to come back that is a piece of peculiar luck.

But to come back to your question; the situation may not be as simple as it seems. We can look, for instance, at Mohammedan countries where the female is articulately devalued and devalued because she endangers the male. From the moment she is born she is a menace to her father, her brother, her husband, and later to her son, because through her they can be dishonoured. But, we do not find in examining the psychology of women in those countries, that they are as insecure as the men; it seems to some extent to be reassuring that you can make that much trouble for that many men. On the other hand, it is exceedingly unreassuring to a man to have these many points of vulnerability in his life, so a rather complicated reversal occurs here. I had a great deal of trouble when I had reasonably feministic young American women anthropologists trying to work on mid-eastern countries, because they assumed that women were treated badly and it was very difficult to focus their attention on the fact that they were looking at a society which was much more psychologically hazardous for men than for women.

FREMONT-SMITH:
Would it not then be asking the wrong question to say 'What does culture do to this particular sex?'

MEAD:
You must always say 'What does it do to both sexes?' Any discussion of one sex without the other is quite useless. You may have a

23

culture which does not verbally discriminate the sexes and has one word for child, say, but even so the social discrimination is there from a very early period. We have no culture that assumes the lack of anatomical sex difference, although we have cultures that ritually relegate human beings to an animal status or that ritually disregard sex for quite a while after birth as far as names are concerned.

Now, if I can leave for a moment this question of the way in which sex differentiation permeates every aspect of social structure, I think it is probably necessary to say here that there is no such thing as the mythical matriarchy that European tradition has constructed. There is no society in which women have the sort of power that men have in most societies. There are societies in which women may nominate for office, there are societies in which they own the houses, there are societies where women are the priestesses or the mediums or the soothsayers, but the nightmare of a female domination that gets conjured up in European folklore is a fantasy. It is parallelled elsewhere —in the Pacific, for instance, by a very widely spread legend of an island of women in which women are able to produce children without the aid of men, and there are large numbers of fantasies in which the men finally break into this society, teach the women how to have children properly and get them under control.

GREY WALTER:
But there is the traditional history of the European matriarchy which is said to have preceded the era of. . . .

MEAD:
We have no suggestion on the basis of anything we have ever been able to examine that there were ever true matriarchies of any sort; as I say, any one of the items that are attributed to a matriarchy may occur separately, but this assumption that there was once a society entirely ruled by women is, as far as we know, a fantasy.

GREY WALTER:
Pure fantasy?

MEAD:
Pure fantasy—so far as we have any reason to judge at present. But the myth of matriarchy has played a very great role in several very important places, in psychoanalytic theory it played a considerable role, and still does; in communism it played a role in Marxian theory by the sheer accident that Engels read an American anthropologist named Morgan (1907), who had been exceedingly

24

impressed by the Iroquois Indians in which the nominating power for chieftainship rested with women.

In constructing a unilateral sequence of evolution on 19th century lines what was done was to start with our civilization and work backwards. Anything we didn't have was earlier and inadequate, so that if you put monogamy and a patriarchally organized society that was patrilocal, patrinomal, patrilineal, patriopotestive and monogamous at the peak, and then you worked back, inevitably you had to have a matriarchal society at one point and group marriage at another. But as far as our present knowledge goes there is no evidence whatsoever for either of these two fantasy institutions.

LORENZ:
The group marriage, I happened to read about that in Russia, was that entirely fantasy?

MEAD:
It is entirely fantasy.

LORENZ:
The group marriage in Samoa, among Polynesians, was entirely fantasy?

MEAD:
Entirely fantasy.

LORENZ:
Oh, I am glad to hear that!

MEAD:
There are various sorts of situations in which, for instance, all the males of a lineage group may have access to their brothers' wives, so that there are various sorts of polygamy and concubinage and special licence, but they do not fall under the head of marriage in the sense that these historical fantasies postulate. It is exceedingly popular at present for commentators, especially European commentators, to describe the United States as a matriarchy. But the United States is a country in which a woman takes her husband's name, moves where he moves, can be legally chastized for not staying where he is, her children take his name, he is responsible for supporting the family and she is not, and so on. I think it is necessary to get rid of this matriarchal daydream at all levels if we are going to be able to consider the question of sex differentiation.

25

ZAZZO:

There are societies where the affiliation can be established only through the mother, the role of the father not yet being known. Perhaps one has no right there to speak of a matriarchy because after all it is a man, the brother of the mother, therefore the uncle, who is responsible for the child. But whether we speak of a matriarchy or not, this fact is very important in the definition of culture: I would like to ask you, therefore, what, in your opinion, is the influence of purely uterine affiliation on the conception of the woman and on her role and importance.

MEAD:

I didn't say all societies were patriarchal, by any means. There are quite a large number of societies which are what we call matrilineal, which means that ties are established through women and that a man inherits from his mother's brother. None of these societies exist at a very simple level—we regard them, on the whole, as an elaboration that is more complicated than the simplest hunting society. In such a society the mother's brother has the power. Power is still in the hands of the male and the fact that it is the mother's brother rather than the father may have important psychological determinants in the constellation of the household, as Malinowski pointed out years ago in the study of the Trobrianders. But it does not change the essential point, that the public power of disposal of property, of chieftainship, and so forth, is in the hands of men. The power goes through women, through your sister instead of through your wife, but it goes from a male to a male.

The only thing I think we can say is that on the whole it is difficult to combine polygamy and matriliny. Why this is so we are not certain, because in patrilineal societies it is quite frequent for women to approve of polygamy and insist upon it; there are many societies in which a woman feels very put upon if she has to conduct a monogamous marriage and will nag and nag her husband into getting her another wife, either to share the onerous duties of sex or bring in the firewood or look after the children or go fishing or whatever. However, when you have a matrilineal society, there is a very strong tendency for what may conceivably be a basic female preference for monogamy to assert itself. Or, you can argue quite differently and say that the tie between the mother and the child is given biologically and that one of the things that human society has had to do is to build up the position of the father, institutionalize it, dramatize it, make it firm and reliable to the extent that the care of the young is dependent upon a stable father. Matrilineal institutions may over-

26

weight the position of the mother and the mother's kin and put the father in a particularly weak role and this may be one reason also why matriliny is less stable. Matriliny tends to yield to patriliny on the whole more easily than patriliny yields to matriliny.

HUXLEY:

This is extremely interesting about matriarchy in the strict sense being pure fantasy; but isn't there a great difference in different societies in the amount of public power and public status accorded to the two sexes? Thus in West Africa you have the queen mothers, though their public role is somewhat overshadowed by the elders. Isn't there a complicated balance, which varies from society to society?

MEAD:

In very simple societies where, for example, there are no buildings of any importance, and there is no political structure for anybody to play a role in, you may have what looks like a very even-handed division. In a very simple food-getting people like the Eskimo, both male and female play absolutely essential economic roles, so that an Eskimo male without a wife is as helpless as an Eskimo woman without a husband. Then you have all the intermediate possibilities from the societies with large harems where women are completely shut off from public life, to the societies, of which West Africa, some Pacific societies, and some American Indian societies are examples, in which women are permitted considerable public roles, sometimes just single individuals as queens or priestesses, and sometimes every woman. Or you may restore even-handedness again as was done in traditional China where although women were confined to the household, they were extraordinarily powerful, so that when modernization started in China these very powerful women moved out and established banks right away. You can sometimes get a measure of the strength that women exercise in various domestic roles by the role that they can play when the barriers are let down and new occupational opportunities are given.

LORENZ:

Was Pearl Buck roughly correct about these things?

MEAD:

Her early book about China is roughly correct about this, I think. The Queen mother, the mother-in-law, had the most enormous power. Every young Chinese girl lived to be a mother-in-law. That was the acme of power. This was reciprocated by the male living for the day when he no longer had any economic or clerical responsibility, so that you had an expectation of maturity roles in which the woman expected to get stronger and stronger while the man expected to retire to a more childlike and protected position. This again is another dimension of the whole picture: women may expect that their position will be enhanced as they grow older, so that their post-menopausal position is one of greater freedom—perhaps even greater than male freedom; on the other hand, they may expect to become less and less desired, desirable or colourful as they get older.

I think, perhaps, I should say here too that there are many students of this subject who feel that the relative safety of women in child-birth today is something that has to be taken into account as a major change in the position and psychological security of the sexes. If you grew up in a society where very many women died in child-birth, so that this was an expected event, and pain was very severe, this permeates the whole position of the girl from the start.

Culture can alter this, however. For instance, in some South African tribes, women are expected to shriek, scream, writhe, and go through the most terrific expressions of agony, and all the little girl children are brought along to watch, so they will know how to have a baby. In other societies women are enjoined to the greatest stoicism, and to utter a single cry would be to proclaim yourself not a woman, and again the little girls are brought along to see that they behave like this. In most of the primitive Pacific island societies where I have worked, and the ones where men are not allowed to witness childbirth, the women are stoical. The men give pantomimes of extreme pain and agony, and have shown me all about childbirth, rolling on the floor and screaming and behaving in a way that no woman under any circumstances in that society has ever behaved. In other words, they either have carried on a memory from some earlier culture that has been perpetuated in the male culture, or this is sheer fantasy behaviour. Now, in this case, you will have young males brought up with a picture of something that happens to females that doesn't happen, and it becomes a component of male psychology and not of female psychology.

One other point about sex roles should be mentioned now, and that is what are the societies which admit transvestism, and of which type. We find societies which do not recognize or admit the pos-sibility of any sexual confusion whatsoever, so that although the spectator interested in constitution might identify a male or female who looked less identifiably male or female than other members of the group, yet the group will have no conception of homosexuality or transvestism, in which case the chances of physical deviation being taken advantage of would be very slight. But there are other societies in which, from the moment the child is born, there are three possibilities: it may be a male, or a female, or a transvestite. The day on which it is born, whether a bird flies over its cradle, the way it drinks its milk the first time, how its teeth come in—any number of such things may be an indicator of whether this child is going to be, as we call it technically in anthropology, a *berdache*. Among many warlike American Indian tribes, for instance, and among the primitive tribes of Siberia, there is both male and female transvestism. Both male and female transvestites have special religious powers, and therefore have an honorific role in the society. The Plains Indians material is, I think, the most vivid, because you have parents, aunts and uncles, grandparents, watching a small boy literally from birth, to find out whether he will be a man or a *berdache*. The role of the *berdache* is completely conventionalized. A man assumes female clothes and is spoken of as 'she' in most of these tribes. He has special activities, such as a go-between in love affairs, or a story-teller on a war party. Interestingly enough, in some of these tribes any sign of female homosexuality will be punished with death. With this expression of anxiety on the part of the adult as to the future social behaviour of the small males a certain number of small boys decides to be transvestites. The whole role is there and they know exactly how to behave, and in turn perpetuate the institution.

FREMONT-SMITH:

Dr. Tigani of the Sudan told me that there is in southern Sudan a tribe where transvestism is part of the social organization, and there are actual marriage ceremonies between males, one dressed as a woman and the other one as a man. He said this needed to be studied in the next few years because the tribe is still relatively isolated, but would not remain so very much longer.

MEAD:

These 'marriages' occur in various parts of the world. We have them among the American Indian Mohaves, with very elaborate rituals of relationship, with complete denial on the part of the male, who is dressed as a woman, of having any male genitals of any sort, and then fake pregnancies, fake deliveries, and fake burial of the fake child which was fake-conceived.

LORENZ:

How far are these transvestites homosexuals?

29

MEAD:

Sometimes they are homosexual (that is, have overt sex relations with members of the same sex), sometimes they are not homosexual. You can have a transvestism that is definitely associated with overt homosexuality, but you can have a transvestism that is disassociated from it in every way.

LORENZ:

I ask this question because in psychiatric practice I came up against two male transvestites and one of them was such a beautiful 'girl' that you were surprised to see 'her'. He said for instance, 'Ich bin eine gute Schwimmerin'—he talked of himself as a female but he was not in the least homosexual: he had a double life, as a man and as a woman. The other was a locomotive driver on the railway, who did exactly the same thing. He had a wife and children in a perfectly normal way and, just as some men go boozing for some days, he changed into a woman for a few days.

HUXLEY:

Margaret, did you say that in the American Indian tribes the boys could opt for what they wanted to do; was it a conscious choice?

MEAD:

Well, it amounts to opting, you see, because people keep testing you out—are you going to be brave enough to be a warrior? If you decide not to be so brave, then your role has been decided for you.

TANNER:

At what age would this occur? At what age is the choice made for the child?

MEAD:

Well, the final choice would be made when you go on your first war-party, which would be early adolescence. Everybody has been saying it for years, you see, but the actual choice comes when there is a request or a need to participate either as a warrior or not as a warrior.

TANNER:

Is there any social stigma or devaluation, when a man opts to be a *berdache*, or by his behaviour on this war-party turns himself into a *berdache*?

MEAD:
He doesn't turn himself into a *berdache*. It isn't that he fails, that he becomes a coward and gets called a *berdache*. He just continually opts not to become a warrior.

ERIKSON:
There is a way of opting by letting the supernatural powers opt for you. If a young man can manage to have an appropriate dream, that dream may be interpreted by those who know dreams as a supernatural suggestion to become a *berdache*. It is like an objective curse, only unconsciously opted. There are also ways of being freed of the curse, and being declared cured by the 'experts.'

MELIN:
In what number do *berdaches* occur?

MEAD:
I've never seen an adequate statistical study. In Siberian tribes there are usually several such persons. Among the Omaha, an American Indian tribe, when I was there, there was only one *berdache* out of 1,500 people. But warfare had ceased, and this particular *berdache* was a man that would have been a homosexual in almost any society—in any society, that is, that selected an extreme degree of feminization for homosexuality. He was the only one left, under conditions of peace, where all the pressures had disappeared.

HUXLEY:
Surely the proportion would never have been more than about five or ten per cent?

MEAD:
I think it was probably never more than five per cent. But it's present as a possibility for every male. It becomes a component in his picture of himself, and this tends to force him into a degree of bravery, or masculinity, that is more extreme than occurs in a society that permits a very wide range of possible roles, including a large number of mild ones.

★   ★   ★

MEAD:
In Professor Zazzo's comments earlier, to which I replied only in part, the question was raised of those societies in which physical paternity is not recognized. I think it is important to emphasize that we do have societies of this sort which are patrilineal. In Aus-

31

tralia societies which are completely patrilineal, in which women leave their own territory to go and live with their husbands, and children grow up within their father's band, nevertheless, have no explicit recognition of physical paternity. (Children are born as a result of spirit action, women going near centres where spirit children are produced.) So that ignorance of paternity and matrilineal ways of reckoning descent do not necessarily occur together in known human society. This, however, does not necessarily compromise the probability that in a much earlier stage of history when there was no knowledge of physical paternity—and I think we must assume such a period—a man attached himself to a woman and her offspring without any recognition that he had any connexion with these children except through the woman. Thus a likely beginning of the family could have been a male wishing to appropriate to himself the attention of a female and being willing to take the children with her. This would not be a matrilineal society, because you would not yet have a form of social organization which is as elaborate as what we mean by matriliny.

FREMONT-SMITH:

It would be very interesting to get Dr. Lorenz to make a comment on this with respect to lower animals, where presumably paternity is not recognized yet where the family certainly is well developed. Would this explanation that Margaret gave fit in with your observations?

LORENZ:

Perfectly satisfactorily.

HUXLEY:

Surely in many cases something quite different happens. In some species of birds, for instance, the male has no parental instinct whatever and does not play any part in brooding or in looking after the young, in others he does not brood but helps to look after the young, and in still others he has completely similar parental instincts to the female. Clearly, there may be parental instincts without any knowledge of the fact of paternity.

MEAD:

Oh, certainly, yes. We have no evidence at present of what might be called a parental instinct in human males but we have the possibility of a protective response to the young of the species. We find this in some monkeys and in apes, where any male will respond to the cry of a very small helpless member of the same species. The present condition in the United States, in which we have the extraordinary change in the expectation of family size, coupled with the young father taking a great deal of care of the human infant, suggests that at present we may be using a biologically-given potentiality of the human male that has not been used in the history of civilization. In very simple societies, such as the Australian aborigines, many South Sea island societies, and some African societies, the male takes a great deal of care of the young infant. But with every society that we have any record of, with the onset of what you call civilization, division of labour, class structure, hierarchies of authority, etc., one of the first things that has happened has been the separation of the human male from his own baby until any point up to two years, four years, six years, twelve years. In some societies he has virtually nothing to do with his son until he is an adolescent. I think one of the things that we may want to discuss here is whether this is not a *condition* of civilization, and whether one of the origins of creativity in males has not been this preventing them from having anything to do with babies.

ZAZZO:
It seems to me that the discussion would be easier if we distinguished between sociability and culture. I think that this emotive reaction, this very primitive communion, is the first element and the very stuff of human sociability. Culture comes afterwards and can integrate or reduce this mode of reaction. Human society has its root in biology thus defined, given the physical debility and the parasitism of the infant. But culture imposes a certain structure, a certain mode of life, which gives to sociability its particular forms. The biological and social contributions in the human being are basically closely interdependent.

HUXLEY:
If you go to biology, it is quite clear that in some mammals, for example bears, the male has no parental instinct or whatever you like to call it, no interest in the young.

LORENZ:
Though in others the reverse is true. For example in all wild *Bovidae* (for instance, cattle) there is a very strict separation of the babies, because male babies play and are taken care of mainly by the bull, the herd bull.

HUXLEY:

So that there can be a complete presence or absence of a parental something: it may be merely the tendency or desire to look after a helpless creature, but it is in essence, biologically speaking, a parental instinct. I should have thought Zazzo was quite right in saying that a man is biologically endowed with a parental instinct or tendency which can be changed—blocked or accentuated—according to the culture in which he lives.

MEAD:

Don't you think that we probably have to assume a period in human evolution when the infants were entirely taken care of by the mother, when the mother found the food for the infant and the male role was restricted to protecting? Certainly, if we use the other primates as an example. . . .

LORENZ:

The trouble is that we don't know the behaviour of anthropoid apes in this respect. Nobody has even tried to observe in captivity how a chimpanzee father behaves to his own baby. He may have much more parental care reactions than a baboon or a Rhesus, in which we know that he only defends the baby in case of extreme need but does not play with it, does not hug it, does not carry it except when he retrieves it from an enemy. We do not know how many 'female' activities a male chimp has, so there is no source of knowledge for our reconstructing how human fathers would behave if left to their infants alone without any cultural influence.

MEAD:

And we have absolutely no material from primitive societies. The important thing to emphasize here is that every primitive society in existence is as old as our own, that they are all the same species of man, that they all depend on shared, learned behaviour, they all have culture. We find great differences of complexity, differences of technology, differences of the size of units that can be integrated, but the sort of evidence that anthropology can produce is evidence on variations possible to human beings *within* culture.

BOWLBY:

I would like to ask a question. Am I right in supposing that there is some agreement amongst us that human males have a parental response to a helpless baby?

34

MEAD:
A protective response.

BOWLBY:
In what way is it suggested that the protective response of the human male is distinguished from the protective response of the human female? It seems to me that in neither sex is there an inherent tendency to direct the response towards their own baby—that is a learned aspect of the response which occurs after birth.

HUXLEY:
But the general tendency may still be inherent.

MEAD:
If we take what we know, say about the behaviour of mother pigs, or mother sheep and goats, there are a very large number of specific responses of the mother to her own infant that are related to the moment and nature of delivery, the smell of the infant, the point at which the infant attaches itself to its mother in lactating and so forth. I agree that this is very poorly explored, but there seems to be a certain amount of suggestion that there are relationships between the mother and the child that she bears that may be of quite a different order from her relationship to all other infants. You can find societies in which a mother doesn't respond to other infants.
A human mother, when she responds to other infants, may be generalizing an identification with her own mother and then learning a female role in her society. Or she may be externalizing or generalizing a specific response to her own young. Similarly the human male may be specializing a general protective response to the young of the species. I think we need to explore this question much further, and explore in terms of, for instance, the effect on maternal acceptance of the child of the use of anaesthesia at delivery.

HUXLEY:·
Then there is your point, Konrád, about the releaser action of certain types of face, the Pekinese and the pug-dog, the little baby face, that seems to stimulate the parental instinct.

LORENZ:
If you are male and observe yourself in your response to a sweet baby, a sweet, helpless baby, I think most of the human race present will agree that our reactions are emotionally, qualitatively, very similar to those of the females. It is exactly the same type of baby

that we find sweet, exactly the same type of baby that we want to help and the only difference is that after a short time we want to put it away again while the female will look after it for days on end. So this is a quantitative and not a qualitative difference. Harping again on my teacher, Hochstetter's, pedantically uttered sentence—'there are no primitive animals, there are only primitive characters: what we call a primitive animal is just one which is rich in primitive characters'—I wonder whether Huxley would agree that we Western whites are particularly rich in unspecialized traits, maybe richer than some of the so-called savages. Maybe, from the evolutionary point of view, we are in a similar situation in comparison to the so-called primitives as man as a whole is to his next relation, the anthropoid apes. Maybe, we are particularly plastic, particularly reticulate, particularly, let's say, hopeful from an evolutionist point of view. Anyhow, I am quite prepared to think that in the primitive characters of male parental care, I myself am more similar to Australians than to Red Indians or others of this type of culture.

MEAD:
I don't think you have any proof of that, Konrad.

LORENZ:
Let it go. If you ask what culture might do to these emotional reactions, of which Professor Zazzo was talking, which I may translate into unlearned or innate reactions, the answer is that culture might very easily suppress them altogether. Then they may live for ages latently in suppression and pop out again the moment they are not tabooed any more and, if I may jump from species psychology very directly to individual psychology, I know that my father had all the hugging instincts and baby-carrying urges which I have myself, but that he simply was too dignified and could not allow himself to do it. I am quite sure that my father was culturally prevented from giving utterance to these, certainly instinctive, urges.

HUXLEY:
There is one final point: one of the most exciting things about recent ethological work is the discovery that there may be super-normal stimuli to innate urges; and so culture may provide a super-normal stimulus which quantitatively increases certain responses. Isn't that what you are saying in different terms?

MEAD:
Yes, quite.

LORENZ:

All baby clothing is an excellent illustration of this.

FREMONT-SMITH:

If I may say one word that is not quite to the point, but because it interests me so much: in trying to think about the problem of international understanding, one asks oneself, where is there a common denominator for all nations and all cultures? One then sees immediately that religion won't do, because the divergencies are already too great; that culture won't do, because the cultural divergencies are already too great, and therefore, one must find something that is more fundamental, from my point of view, than religion, more fundamental than culture, and so I thought that, well, we must go to the biological level. And then, in going to the biological level for the common denominator, what I came to was the parental concern for their very young, which is the common denominator in all human species. I know there are exceptions where they throw them away and where they may destroy them. Nevertheless, no race would survive if there were not very deep parental concern for their very young from the instant of birth on, either through actual parents, or parent surrogates.

MEAD:

But while it is true that no race survives without some concern for the young, yet we have no reason to believe that there have not been many human groups that lost such a concern, or failed to use it in some way, and didn't survive. The Mundugumor, for example, of the Sepik River area of New Guinea, were a non-viable social group, and had probably only existed in the form we knew for five or six generations. They went down at once before contact with the Europeans. It was an extraordinarily weak society and it is an accident of history that they were ever recorded. I think we have to consider that there have been many such small—and large—civilizations, so that we cannot postulate in human behaviour a biological basis which is automatically self-preserving. We have to envisage the possibility of human culture building a superstructure which is non-viable as well as one that is viable.

HUXLEY:

This is very like the old dilemma, which is really meaningless, of which is more important, heredity or environment. The answer is *neither*, because both are necessary. Similarly in man you've got to

37

have the innate urges and you have also got to have the cultural environment to bring them out in a viable way.

LORENZ:

And culture may do everything analogous to mutation. Just as you have lethal mutation, you may develop a lethal culture.

ERIKSON:

May I go back for a moment to the cultural evaluation of masculine and feminine? It is my impression, and this is a question to Margaret Mead, that in America it was primarily the generation of young soldiers, coming back from the second World War, which made it seem permissible for a man to take care of a baby. This had something to do with the fact that for them there was no more question that they were men; they had been soldiers, they had fought, and they had taken care of the whole nation. They could do what the women could do without being called feminine or effeminate. On the other hand, it is very difficult to keep young clinicians from calling a man who is less a man than most men 'feminine' in a case history. I try to teach that, for example, a marked homosexual does not have a 'feminine' bearing but an 'effeminate' one, often a mocking caricature of femininity. In the same way, in clinical histories a woman is called more 'masculine' if she is less of a woman, when she really is more 'mannish', often again to the point of obvious mockery. The evaluation of the two sexes seems to be polarized in such a way that if you get a little less of one you automatically assume in your evaluation that there is a little more of the other. Do you think this is the case in other cultures also, Margaret?

MEAD:

Well, I would agree that there is a tendency to evaluate as feminine the male who plays less than the particular masculine role that a given society demands. In very many societies women and children are grouped together, with the male as the final point that children can reach, that sometimes menopausal women can almost reach, and that women in a reproductive stage cannot possibly reach. I should say that there is another tendency in most societies to regard plusses, that is the woman who is *more* intelligent, *more* active, *more* skilled than the average woman, as masculine, and the tendency to regard the man who is *less* strong, *less* skilled, *less* intelligent, as feminine (see, for example Franck & Rosen's, 1949, tests of masculinity and femininity). You do, of course, get odd sorts of things. For instance, in Bali, the ideal for both sexes is a kind of sexlessness.

38

The ideal man looks as much like a woman as a man can look and the ideal woman looks as much like a man as a woman can look, and the disliked and disapproved-of types are the woman with large breasts and the hairy man with large muscles. When the Balinese make a picture of the disliked and disapproved and death-dealing aspects of life they make the witch who has both the extreme male secondary sex characters and the most extreme female ones, with masses of body hair and great pendulous breasts. But there seems to be a general tendency to regard the minus position as female and the plus position as male in a great number of societies.

I think, perhaps, the next point that ought to be dealt with is the question of the devaluation of each sex. You often find in human culture a very high valuation placed on femininity or a very high valuation placed on masculinity in the simplest terms, often in terms of the primary genitalia particularly because of their association with reproduction. In a large part of the Pacific centring around New Guinea there is an assumption that women, in terms of their biological capacities to produce children, have the greater power, and that men, to equal the women, must imitate, fictionalize, ritua-lize and construct cultural replicas of that power. This is expressed in a large number of ways; for instance the men build great men's houses, which they call wombs, they go through elaborate ceremonies of giving birth to the initiate so that when the boys are a certain age they will be taken over by the men and fed on the men's blood, which then makes them the children of the men. Up to that point they have had the blood of their mothers and the blood of their mothers' brothers (who are the uterine relatives and belong to the same blood-relation-group), but then the men cut their arms, put blood on coconuts, feed it to the initiates and the initiates are now the men's children. In a large number of these ceremonies the entire ritual is a way of asserting that the men are really the creators of the children; that they, not the women, are the makers of men. This takes all sorts of forms, such as imitations of menstruation among the men, with elaborate cutting of the phallus, because they say women are fortunate, they menstruate every month, they are able to get rid of the bad blood within them; but poor unfortunate males have no way to menstruate, so they create a substitute menstruation. This is the more striking, because in so many parts of the world menstruation is fraught with great fear and a great aversion.

In Europe we find virtually the exact opposite of this position, with male achievements being extremely conspicuous. This is so in any high civilization where there is a superstructure of cultural invention in the hands of males; where men build temples, roads,

39

boats, aeroplanes, supreme courts, parliaments. It is evident to the growing boy and girl that what men do is important and what women do is less important, and in this case you have a devaluation of feminine biological capacities in favour of a high valuation of male capacities. The reason it is necessary to emphasize this particularly is that so much psycho-analytic theory is derived from the European position and has assumed that the natural position of the female is to envy the male. This is very often explained in terms of nursery behaviour, but if we take the whole of human achievement into account it is possible to find situations where male achievement is not high and then female achievement may look very large. But we have no society in which female public achievement is such that there is a denigration of the male because the female is able to do so much publicly; that is really the crucial point about the non-existence of real matriarchy.

We then face the whole question of the way in which the actual anatomical differences between a small boy and a small girl and other people's response to them will influence their picture of their sex role. It is customary to emphasize that the male sexuality is conspicuous and the female is inconspicuous and hidden. But this again can be altered culturally. Take, for example, a society in which little girls are told they are probably pregnant, in which every time a two-year-old little girl passes older people, somebody hits her on the abdomen and says, 'Got a baby in there?' So in Bali, little girls between two and three walk with a 'pregnant' posture and this is quite regardless of whether or not their mothers are pregnant at the moment. Everybody teases them about being pregnant, and in such a case, of course, there is a very early emphasis by the culture on the procreative reproductive role of the female. In other societies, little girls may be dressed in a way that will completely denigrate their femininity.

Among the Iatmul of the Sepik River, little girls are dressed in a very feminine way and boys are dressed more like girls than like boys and it is impossible for an outside observer to tell a boy or a girl apart. Even if you look at them sideways, or look at a moving picture, or analyse their behaviour, you think the boys are girls. On the other hand, among the Manus of the Admiralty Islands, the people I was working with last year, it is impossible to tell the little girls and little boys apart because one thinks all the little girls are little boys. This is primarily a question of posture and stance, which in turn is cultivated by the behaviour of the adults. Among the Iatmul, boys are classed with women, boys are allowed to mourn as women mourn. Grown men cannot mourn under any circumstances, and the one thing that little boys love to play at is mourning. After they have announced that they have completely forgotten what it was like to go with their mothers to mourn, they will, if given toys, continually play at mourning games. Thus the society groups boys with women in its response to them and its expectations from them and there is in boys a feminine stance and posture which has to be altered in adult life. In Manus, on the other hand, which is an exceedingly masculine society, in which women are more or less assimilated to male stereotypes in any event, little girls look and act and move like little boys.*

The cultural expectations can thus have a tremendous effect in emphasizing one aspect or the other of the potential behaviour of the child. There are some societies in which the little baby girl is dressed up at six months with ear-rings and great big rings in her nose and a floppy grass skirt, every man that comes along tickles her and flirts with her and plays with her until femininity is very highly emphasized. Bali is a case where there is enormous emphasis in early childhood on the difference between the male and female genitals. From morning to night there are adjectives which mean 'pretty' for a girl, and 'handsome' for a boy. Adults do a great deal of patting their children's genitals saying 'Pretty, pretty, pretty', or 'Handsome, handsome, handsome'. It is a society where there is no doubt whatsoever as to which sex one belongs to. There is enormous ease about other kinds of sex characteristics, but always with this great and very early identification of the self as belonging to one sex rather than the other. There are societies, for example, many near-Eastern countries, in which small males have pictures taken naked, where there is a tremendous emphasis on maleness from very early days so that masculinity is played up well beyond the

*TANNER:
I can most heartily corroborate this statement. Dr. Schwartz and Dr. Mead took somatotype photographs of Manus children last year and I have been examining these. When I first examined the pictures (before this meeting) I was at once struck by the extreme resemblance of girls to boys, an impression which was shared by the other people, both skilled at somatotyping and otherwise, to whom I showed the pictures. So marked was this impression that I found myself searching for signs of a short penis in the girls' photographs, involuntarily thinking it must be hidden in photographic shadow. Certainly without inspection of the genitalia it is impossible to differentiate the little girls from the little boys, though this is easy enough in W. European and American children. Since there is very little actual difference in measurements and proportions before about age nine, the sex difference is presumably conveyed by posture, attitude and facial appearance (one can tell a male without looking at the hair) and in the Manus children both girls and boys resemble European boys in these respects. It may be worth adding that the pictures of adults show a considerably higher degree of mesomorphy, on average, both for men and women, than one sees in American and West European groups.

41

point at which the child would biologically be prepared to exhibit it.

Here again we have an enormous range and I think the only problem for us is to realize how much variation is possible and how much the sense of sex difference can be accentuated or muted by the society. There is some evidence that girl babies a few months old know difference in sex—certainly by the time they can roll over—and that we can recognize a differentiation in the behaviour of girl babies towards men and women. But on the other hand, human behaviour can probably be so patterned that these differences in behaviour can be held in check right up to puberty, We find societies in which the response of males to females as such can be delayed until a very late date. I would mention present day Australia as an outstanding example, with delayed courtship behaviour in adolescence and the tendency to keep schoolboys and schoolgirls in a relatively sexless state till rather late.

I am purposely dealing here only with the social patterning and not yet bringing in what may be innate stages of development. I want, if possible, to have a sort of interplay between Erikson and myself when we come to dealing with what look like universals in children's stages of psychosexual development and so I must clear away first the very obvious social patterning which will speed up or retard sex consciousness.

INTERVAL

MEAD:

I think in the amount of time that we have left we should finish discussing the extent to which we have a universal differentiation between roles of men and women, which in turn become operative in the learning process of boys and girls. It is very important to emphasize that if to be a man is strong, then the child that is weak is not a man, the child that is strong is more of a man, etc. If to be a female is to burst into tears, then if you are a non-crier, you are that less female, and among the Iatmuls, for instance, in New Guinea, not to be able to cry on demand is one of the most terrible things that can happen to a woman. It is far worse than having the wrong figure, because crying is something that is expected of every woman. Every time there is a death, all the women in the group gather together and cry, and the pressure is enormous. I might say that I am reasonably easily suggestible and I usually find it quite possible to cry whenever it is appropriate, and often when it isn't, but in that tribe, I took a large onion, cut it into little bits, put it in my handkerchief, went to a mourning festival and rubbed onion on my eyes, and didn't have one tear. The pressure and the sense of tenseness everywhere is so great that all the people who have the slightest counter-suggestibility to crying are unable to cry.

Any sort of trait that is sex-identified in a given society has this sort of effect. Among the Arapesh, women do the carrying because women's heads are stronger. That means that for a man to carry a load on his head would be to become to that degree a feminine personality. At the limit, however, there is still a set of universals. There is no society that we know of in which men are not stronger than women at the point of strongest work, where men are not expected to drag down the great log for a lost canoe, to hunt the large animal, to go to war, to do the things that involve the greatest display of strength. This does not mean that in many societies women don't do things that men do in others, but the *ratio* is always preserved. So that the picture of strength is systematically presented to boys as compared with girls.

There are, however, some rather striking variations even to this picture. The position of Russian peasants is an example, where the woman is an exceedingly strong person physically, and where there is a certain amount of evidence to suggest that wife-beating in Russia was not a form of sadism but was a necessity. The only way in which the Russian peasant male equalled the Russian peasant female was with a whip in his hand, and society provided the whip. There are also very marked differences in the extent to which the women are smaller than men. All the same this physical difference in strength between the sexes and its social implications survives right through the world until the present stage of automatic machinery. Now, however, we are moving into a period of automatic machinery where we are getting rid of the relationship between physical effort and result, so that you can now press the button on an ack-ack gun, or press the button on a giant lever. The association between sheer physical strength and work productivity is no longer real.

However, in every society that we know anything about at present those things which are regarded as most worth doing are assigned to males. Again there are variations: female goddesses, female priestesses, females taking over almost any function except the exceedingly energetic ones, but when this happens, then these occupations are no longer the most highly valued ones. When we read about an ancient society in which there were female priests, we read of this from the point of view of our own society in which women are not in general allowed to be members of the clergy. Then we tend to say that if the society had female priestesses, these people must have given a very high position to women—which isn't necessarily true

43

at all. The one thing that we can say consistently is that in every society we know anything about, whatever men do is important, and if men dress dolls, dressing dolls is important, if men make baskets, basket-making is an important activity and if women make baskets it is not as important an act. If men cook, it is because cooking is sacred—if women cook, it is because cooking is low-grade.

If you survey the cultures of the world you find curing can be a woman's activity or a man's activity, being a soothsayer can be male or female, making baskets can be male or female, weaving can be male or female, dressing dolls can be male or female, gossiping can be male or female, shopping can be male or female. Almost any sort of activity is interchangeable at this rather superficial occupational kind of level. But if you then look at the evaluation placed on that activity, it is valued when it is male disproportionately to the way it is valued when it is female. It doesn't mean that basket-making by women is disapproved of, but, if a man makes a basket people say, 'Why are you making a basket, that's something that women do! What do you want to do that sort of thing for?' and it is less than, say, making pottery, which is something the male does in that particular society. This seems to be, to date, and in the societies we know anything about, a universal. Now it seems rather difficult to explain it on the simple historical ground that in every society women were bound by childbearing to the home, and by breast-feeding, with no means of locomotion for the baby before you had baby carriages and feeding bottles. It is possible to say that women were inevitably bound to certain tasks such as cooking, and that left men free for all the elaborative tasks, and that historically these would therefore be very conspicuous and important advancements in the life of the society, and that they became more valued. That possible interpretation is one that some people prefer as a hypothesis.

An alternative hypothesis can be derived from the circumstance that boys and girls are both initially cared for by women. Although there are primitive societies where men take a great deal of care of little babies, they can't feed them, so they are always handing them back to the mother to be fed. They can't take them off on long trips. The tie between the breast-feeding mother, or the wet nurse and the baby has been pretty absolute up to the present, so that children of both sexes are brought up and cared for by a parent of one sex. If we take this as a primary condition to date, though not an inevitable one, we can examine the whole process by which the mother treats the children of both sexes differently and the child identifies with the parent. A girl is identifying with someone who

44

smells like herself, moves like herself, feels like herself, and treats her as if she were like herself. On the other hand, the boy is continually given the task of differentiating himself away from the mother and stressing his behaviour as different from what he sees her as being, a reproductive creature. It is possible that an extra urge towards achievement may be given boys in the course of this sort of upbringing, which would not occur otherwise. In other words, there may be no innate urge to achievement in males that is different from an innate urge to achievement in the females, but the conditions of nurture are such that they are differently developed.

Perhaps one of the most fruitful lines of discussion in this group will be the way that a biological potentiality, which is either the same for both sexes and differentiated by upbringing, or different for both sexes and further emphasized or de-emphasized by upbringing, will give us an area of possible intervention in human development. This is also a point of great potential cross-fertilization between ethology, for instance, and cultural study. An exploration of the extent to which children of both sexes have always been reared by their mothers and the meaning of this very close tie might be one of the best approaches that we could have to our subject.

ERIKSON:

As to achievement in males—that even goes for the *berdaches* you mentioned earlier. They became cooks—often famous cooks. A woman could cook, but a *berdache* had the chance to become an artist in cooking. Women could embroider, but a *berdache* became a famous embroiderer. Whether they actually did cook better, I would not know.

LORENZ:

That is the question I wanted to put. Is it not that men—as a universal rule—are slightly more creative in inventions, and slightly more exploratory than girls are, even when they are quite small children? I was always intrigued with the fact that all little boys go for mechanical toys and girls don't, not even when the adored elder brother does so. There is no absolute rule—there are girls who play with mechanical toys—but I think that I see a slight dimorphism in the exploratory behaviour in boys and girls, that boys are more interested in mechanics. In primitive man, at the palæolithic level, experimentation of this kind must play a very large role. I suppose the way in which the first stone implements were invented was by just this kind of play, which you see in monkeys, too, and in apes.

45

Well, here again it is so difficult to separate the social features because if you take a society which is based on the horse and horsemanship is an important element for men, you will find that little girls do not pay as much attention to the horses. If it were possible to look at such a society, say 500 years ago, it would be quite clear that the association between the male and the horse was a sensible one that had all sorts of psychological concomitants—the man was active, he rode, and the female did not want to go long distances, she was afraid of this great big animal, and so forth. But today in the urban United States, horses have become a female interest as men have taken over the motor car, and furthermore there is now a slight indication that motor cars are becoming female, while aeroplanes become male.

If you look at this closely you begin to wonder whether it is not some *ratio* of degree of activity that must be preserved. Thus it may be that males are not universally more exploratory than females, but that a male-female harmony is achieved in some way by an accentuation to a higher level in the male than the female in any one particular group. We can find societies in which the little boys are extraordinarily non-exploratory, where they are very passive and quiet. In Bali, it is a tremendous effort to get the little boys out of the home and all sorts of rewards are given—for example an enormous great big hatchet-like knife that they can wear in their belts. Each little boy is given a water-buffalo or an ox that is his own, if he will only go and ride it and care for it. The whole society is trying to make the male a little bit more adventurous and a little more exploratory than the female. And after all these pressures have been exerted, he *is* a little more exploratory. However, in most societies the boys between, say, six and twelve are infinitely more curious and brighter than little girls, so that in most societies when I go in to work, I work with little boys. They are three times as interesting, they have got a lot of intellectual curiosity, where girls, relatively speaking, are just little bores. They have already taken on the domestic attitudes—they talk just like their mothers, they have less freedom of the imagination of any sort.

That is true in most societies, but not all. Among the Tchambuli where the women have taken on a great many of the functions that are male in most societies, the little girls were the more enterprising. It was the little girls who would go with me to explore something, who became the informants on language, while the little boys were moping about all by themselves at home. That was a society in which there had been a marked reversal of roles, which conceivably

46

was also psychologically expensive. Our hypotheses either have to be that the male is more exploratory, in all circumstances, than the female, or that for any society to be viable a higher degree of male exploration must be maintained whether both sexes display this character at a very high or a very low level.

GREY WALTER:

It is obviously necessary for an explanation to include the biological difference between men and women, but do you, yourself, think this is a sufficient one, for the observed asymmetry in their social tasks and achievement rating?

MEAD:

I think that is an unanswered question. I am surveying what material we have from existing conditions in existing societies, and trying to present the questions that are raised by it. Most societies want girls to be a little less active than boys, for instance, to sit usually in a slightly more demure fashion, to enclose the body more— there are many varieties of this expectation—to be at home at night, or to wear more clothes, or to behave in a more modest fashion. In spite of great variety these cultural expectancies are remarkably consistent. It is possible to interpret this historically, or to interpret it as a way of adapting girls to their future roles as women. And/or it is possible to say that at the age of two, or three, or four, the human female is less exploratory, less active and less extended than the male. All three of these statements may be true. But these, I think, are the sorts of hypotheses that are suggested by the material. I am not arguing for one as compared with the other at the moment. I am just trying to present them.

ZAZZO:

I would like to make three remarks.

The first, in connexion with what Margaret Mead said about differences between men and women of a physical order (strength, height, etc.) which determine differences of a psychological order. It is quite obvious that for the sexual characteristics there is no question of all or nothing and as regards the characteristics of which you have been speaking, especially height, there is a considerable overlap in the statistical distribution of heights in men and women. It seems to me, however, interesting from the psychological point of view that whatever our physical or individual strength and whatever our height, we keep to the psychological stereotype of our sex. A masculine individual who is smaller and weaker than average will

47

in general keep, nevertheless, to the masculine stereotype, that of the 'stronger' sex.

The second remark concerns the valuation of tasks and the attribution of social tasks to the man or to the woman. Don't you think that in order to make some progress in the understanding of these problems it is necessary to take into account the mode of life, the economic structure and the geographical conditions? A nomadic people does not have the same attitude towards children, nor does it have the same valuation of tasks as a sedentary or agricultural people or as a society based on real estate. I think it is necessary to take these factors into account in order to understand the social valuation of tasks, the distribution of tasks between man and woman, and also in order to understand the importance accorded to the child. In a society where inheritance does not exist the child is differently valued.

Third remark: for some years we have been making a systematic study in my laboratory of differences between sexes, and we have looked for the origin of these differences as far back as possible in childhood. Well, these differences appear very early: at the age of two years they are already considerable. When restandardizing Gesell's 'baby tests' on a French population we discovered that boys from the age of two years, perhaps even before, are more advanced than girls in the tests of motor co-ordination; that boys from the age of two to three years are more advanced than girls in all the tests of spatial organization. On the other hand, as soon as language comes in, girls show for several aspects of spoken or written language a certain superiority over the boys. I won't labour the point. Two categories of factors seem to come into the psychological differentiation between sexes: factors of physiological differentiation, which are often very weak and noticeable very early; they are amplified by social factors, in the first place through examples given by the father and the mother.

MEAD:

I think the only thing that I need to say at this point is that I am not arguing at all against the possibility of universal differences between the sexes. I am trying to present the material from the anthropological field that creates a framework within which we can look at these differences. We only have information on children's language in a very limited number of societies but in every one that I know, the girls are more precocious than the boys in linguistic behaviour to an extent which is measurable.

As to the question of a correlation between stages of technological

48

development and the role of the sexes, and the role of the child within these differently developed societies, when we examine these carefully we do not find a very close correspondence. There are agricultural societies in which the aged are treated very badly, and agricultural societies in which they are treated very well, even though there is the nice farm for them to stay on in each case. There are nomadic societies in which the aged are treated with enormous care even though they are a drain on the economy of the whole community and in which the old men remain the great power in the group, and there are nomadic societies in which the aged have no power whatsoever. So that, although the technology and the stage of economic development will always be a limiting factor in the situation, we have no material to date to show that the technology is consistently important in determining which sex roles or which attitudes towards children will occur.

BUCKLE:
I think perhaps we need to remember that some of the moulding influences are mythological ones, not merely social, geographical and so on. I wonder about this myth of the matriarchal society—just where does it occur, in what kind of cultures, is it a male myth or a female myth, and how does it influence this whole question of the predominance of the male?

MEAD:
There are almost no female myths, as far as we know, which is a very curious thing. Of course it is also something that is very difficult to prove, because one always finds mythology already there when one arrives in a primitive society and women may be the principal transmitters. In many societies women tell the tales, but to date, most of the analysis that has been done on folk tales suggests that there are a very limited number of female myths, and that when they occur they do not spread. Occasionally you may have a myth that could be regarded as a female myth—Bluebeard, I think is one. The Bluebeard story could be regarded as a female fear and it does not diffuse easily. It is a French tale and the French have been one of the most active people in diffusing mythology all over the world; they have human relations with native peoples everywhere, they tell stories to the people, and usually French tales spread. But Bluebeard just didn't spread. On the other hand, the two most widespread myths in the world are The Magic Flight and The Toothed Vagina—both embodying male fears. These spread with remarkable facility.

D   49

So on the whole we do not think that very many myths are female myths, but whether females are not fantasy builders or simply have not been in a position to build fantasies, we are not quite sure. I think that the matriarchy, the island of women, this whole set of stories are male myths, although in their secondary forms, they may give aid and comfort to some European feminists.

TANNER:

I want to come back, if I may, to Lorenz' question as to whether the little boy was not naturally more exploratory than the little girl. The point I want to make is rather a general one. There is, on average, a difference in physique between males and females that appears considerably before puberty. We have to get it quite clear as to what we mean by maleness and femaleness—there are changes which occur at puberty to make somebody who is prepubescent into male or female, but there are also other non-genital differences between girls and boys existent before puberty, and these may not be anything to do with post-puberty maleness and femaleness, but something which is separate and can best be looked at in a different way. To be concrete, let us think of physique in terms of Sheldon's somato-types. The distribution of somatotypes of little boys and of little girls is in fact different—there is more endomorphy on average in little girls and more mesomorphy (nothing to do with postpubescent sex character) in little boys. Therefore, if the exploratory relation-ship is linked to a basic physique which is present in x per cent. of males, and less than x per cent. of females, this will of itself make little boys on average more exploratory. Whether one can call this a sex difference or not I don't know—this is a matter of the use of words.

FREMONT-SMITH:

As to little girls tending to be more fat than boys, at an early age, that could be for cultural reasons. If the mothers are feeling a bit guilty about having borne a little girl who is going to be in a derogated position all her life, they may have overfed the little girl; we know that obesity in children is likely to be a response of maternal over-com-pensation. So there is a possible psychosocial basis for there being on average more little fat girls than little fat boys.

TANNER:

You would have to extend your explanation to cover the muscu-larity of boys as well, which gets a little difficult. I think this raises

50

genetical questions too. I would presume that there is a balance existing between males and females to maintain this quantitative difference in physique as between the two, and there must be some evolutionary forces acting to maintain it that way. On the one hand it probably is advantageous from an evolutionary point of view to keep a large amount of variability in physique in a population, but it may also be advantageous to have as many muscular active mesomorphic males as possible if you are defending territory. When primate reproduction appears, the female is immobilized for a considerable period, is not able to move from one place to another with the same ease as the male, and is not able to fight for considerable periods. In that case it might be advantageous to push over on to the female the less-useful-for-moving-about characteristics of physique, but nevertheless to preserve these. Though a multi-factorial system, it would act like a balance, I think, because the mechanism couldn't go too far; that is you couldn't get absolutely no mesomorphs among the females, or no endomorphs amongst the males, because then you would lose the variability and that would pull back the system again to where it was before.

ERIKSON:

In general, would it be fair to say, Margaret, that you started with extreme examples and you worked then toward this formulation: there are certain given sex differences which in any culture are elaborated into a certain *ratio*. This ratio rests on many conflicting necessities, one of them being the survival of the young. I would stress that by survival we do not understand merely the first year, as such. In the first year the foundation is created for a baby to become a functioning person, including a parent later on. In other words, survival in a human setting does not mean just to bring up a baby for its own sake and lifetime, as it were, but to bring up somebody who will have the preconditions of becoming a parent later on and a creator of generations to come.

I don't know whether I am the only anxious one in this group, but I felt increasingly anxious when you spoke of the arbitrary changes that are taking place, because I constantly think of what is going to happen to the children. In primitive systems, or at any rate in those which have survived, we are aware of a certain self-correction which establishes a workable ratio, and which does not only depend on what Professor Huxley called the super-normal stimuli bringing out innate virtues. There must be, especially in women, certain correctives, which resist such super-normal stimuli in order to safeguard psychological survival.

51

INHELDER :

As a matter of information I should like to put a question to Margaret Mead, Jim Tanner and Zazzo: what do we know actually about the age of acquisition of walking and, in some cases, of swimming? Are there significant differences between the sexes even for these fundamental co-ordinations, or do these differences not go beyond the normal distribution curves characteristic of individual differences?

MEAD :

Well, I want to go tomorrow into the question of these differences in the young, having sketched out first the adult differences in role that may be important. I would say that here again you find the basic difference that the boy and the girl both learn their motor behaviour from their mother. So, if we find a difference in any given culture between the boys' and the girls' motor behaviour it still does not tell us that it is innate and not learned. To answer such a question we need also the situation where the reverse occurs. In Manus, for example, both boys and girls learn their motor behaviour from their fathers to a very large extent and you have very high motor mobility in both boys and girls, with the girls showing enormously precocious motor behaviour. The possibility exists that there may be a systematic difference in French children, such as Professor Zazzo finds, but not until we do studies of cultures in which children are taught by women, by men, by older children, etc., can we be sure that there are genuine universal sex differences, although I am personally inclined to believe that such exist.

* * *

MEAD :

Let me begin today's session by saying that I am still presenting material on adult sex differences as they may be mediated to children, for the present begging the question as to how far they are biologically determined and how much they are culturally arranged, though emphasizing the cultural arrangement. This morning I want to take up two or three points that are a good deal closer to the biological level, and first I want to ask Jim Tanner a question. What happened to the longer arms of boys than girls? I thought you were going to talk about them yesterday, or have they become submerged in the mesomorphic-endomorphic difference we discussed?

TANNER :

I don't think they have. What Margaret is referring to is the fact that the forearm in the male is considerably longer relative to the upper arm or any other part of the body one cares to take than it is in the female. The data, of course, are only on American and West European adults and children so we don't know whether this is a universal finding. I rather suppose so, all the same.

HUXLEY:
There is an overlap in the male and female distribution, I take it?

TANNER:
Certainly. This greater relative forearm length is present from birth onwards. The mechanism of it is that the growth rate of the male forearm is slightly greater throughout the whole growing period than that of the female forearm. This is probably true of the circumference of the forearm also relative to the other parts of the body though this isn't quite so well documented. There are various other similar differences, as, for example, in the length of the index finger. In the female the second metacarpal is longer relative to all the other metacarpals. That again is first visible very early—in fact, in foetal life; so that it is not a secondary sex difference in the sense that we usually speak of them.

There are three ways in which the male/female physical differences may come about. Some are caused by hormone action at puberty; others, such as the longer legs of the male, come about simply because the male goes on growing for about two years longer than the female and since relative to the rest of the body the legs are growing fastest just before puberty, therefore, they end up relatively longer. Thirdly, a very few dimensions just grow faster all the time right from the start, in one sex or the other, which is the case for the forearm.

HUXLEY:
The difference in arm proportion might help to explain why girls on the whole don't seem to be able to throw a baseball or cricket ball so well as boys.

GREY WALTER:
What order of difference is there in the arm lengths?

TANNER:
It would, I think, be around eight to ten per cent.

GREY WALTER:
I should have thought that a shorter lever might match their weight better for cricket balls.

MEAD:

We might come back later to this difference in the arms in connexion with exploratory and other activity of the male in relation to the outer environment. But I want to discuss first the difference in type of work, or utilization of energy, in males and females. All sorts of investigators have commented that on the whole the male works with spurts of energy and is better at work demanding spurts than a female, who is in turn better than males at slow repetitious monotonous tasks. Gesell and Ilg (personal communication) say that they find this for children as well. However, a culture can reverse it. We have a good deal of material, for instance, on the behaviour of Czech factory workers, who seem to have a high tolerance of monotonous work, correlated with apparently a very high amount of day-dreaming that makes the monotonous work possible. Among my Arapesh people, in New Guinea, where the women do the carrying and where they say the women's heads are so strong, women do virtually no handwork whatsoever. They do heavy work with the body and come home totally exhausted and sit exhausted, exactly as the men do. In Bali, we have a different sort of reversal in that Balinese men hardly go in for spurts at all and have very poor lifting power. But both men and women have good carrying power if a load is placed on their heads, and Balinese men work exactly the way women do with a monotonous, repetitious, dreamy quality. Normally, the Balinese male does not develop heavy muscles, but if he goes to work as a coolie and works for Europeans he develops his muscles just like anyone else, so that there was a small group of males in Bali who looked like he-men, whereas the rest of the population, who had not been exposed to this particular heavy work, had a smooth feminine appearance. Bali is one of the conspicuous instances, I think, of the extent to which culture can modify what looks like a significant difference.

HUXLEY:

What about the sculpture and painting in Bali? Isn't that done almost entirely by men?

MEAD:

Yes, it is done by men, but when a man is carving in Bali, he will use only the absolutely necessary muscles, with the rest of the body uninvolved. In contrast, the Iatmul people, who work entirely in enormous spurts of energy, never do anything except with maximum exertion. They don't believe in doing any work at all until they are in an absolute fury; the only way a woman gets her husband to do any work is to insult him all night long at the top of her voice; or one part of the community insults the other half—'you never caught a crocodile—you never will catch a crocodile, your ancestors didn't catch any crocodiles, you are non-crocodile catchers', and that goes on for about a week. Then the insulted group gets angry enough to go and kill some crocodiles. The whole of male behaviour is based on these enormous spurts. When Iatmul carve the whole body is involved and they get tired very quickly; films demonstrate the enormous over-use of every part of the body. The women work slowly and monotonously and don't share in this big spurt. I think that this sex-differentiated behaviour may be important in conveying to the small child what it is to be male and female, and it is interesting that the Arapesh and the Mundugumor both have failed to differentiate in energy use and both have failed also to differentiate between males and females in personality in general.

LORENZ:
Which of these two people are the river people in New Guinea?

MEAD:
The Mundugumor are the river people who are cannibals and have a system where they change sex-descent each generation. The women are tall and masculine. Their size can be somewhat attributed to the fact that they have all the food; they do all the fishing and they eat what they like before they come into the village. The Arapesh are people where both men and women are mild and parental in behaviour. They also live in New Guinea, about 50 miles away. (See Mead, 1935, 1949 for description of these tribes.)

Now, another dimension of somewhat the same sort that I think is worth considering is the difference in climax structure in the life of the male and the life of the female. The female's life is a series of irreversible events enacted inside her own body which once enacted cannot be denied. First, menstruation, rupture of the hymen, birth, and finally menopause all are irreversible events. Female life moves through a series of indubitable natural climaxes with a rhythm that is internally determined.

From time to time there have been attempts to establish periodicities in males (Hersey, 1931). They have never been controlled adequately in relation to the periodicities in the males' wives and I think there is a reasonably good possibility that they are merely responses in the males to an extreme periodicity in the wives. In some societies this is institutionalized completely, so that when a wife is segregated at menstruation, the husband has to do all the

55

housework and take care of the children, so that you have a periodicity in the life of the male which is at least as irritating as the seclusion of the females concerned.

DE SAUSSURE:

Have you been able to observe correlations between rhythmic work and collective work? When the work is collective is it more rhythmic? When it is rhythmic is it more frequently accompanied by singing than when it is done in spurts? Have individuals who work in a more rhythmic way a tendency to work collectively rather than individually? And on the other hand, when they work individually do they sing while they work?

MEAD:

I don't think we can make any statement about that. It has never really been systematically investigated, although there were some early speculative statements about the relationship between rhythm and work. But I think the problem of whether a male or female rhythm is used all the way through in a society may be more pertinent than the relationship between the individual and the collective.

INHELDER:

To what extent does culture determine the rhythm activity/rest characteristic of the daily individual cycle? Are there cultures where the maximum activity is found in the early hours of the morning, others towards midday or in the evening?

MEAD:

It is possible to find almost every sort of difference in this. There are societies where there are great spurts of work early in the morning, where conceivably the late risers suffer. There are societies where people get up very slowly and organize their approach to any kind of work very gradually. There are people who are very responsive to changes of the wind or changes of the moon and others will plod along at just the same rate, paying little attention to shifts in seasons.

ERIKSON:

How about precision?

MEAD:

I think all the material we have on precision comes from our own society and most of it was work done in the last war. One study was made in which they found women who did fine embroidery were more reliably precise than men watchmakers at a very fine crafts-man's job. I think it is probably important that the watchmaker works with external materials which he is adapting to each other with a very high degree of precision, but the woman who is doing delicate embroidery is still working more with her own body.

FREMONT-SMITH:
It seems to me 'own body' needs to be defined a bit more. This is really a question of whether your own body is using the whole limb or the peripheral fingers, because no matter how external the objects are that the watchmaker is working with, he has got to move his hands and his fingers to do the work.

MEAD:
Both people are working with their fingers, but I think the woman handles the needle much more as a part of her own body than is the case with the man and his tools. The girl does more things with her own body, her body is the theatre on which events are played out, so that if you have a thing like a needle, the way in which the girl uses it will differ from the way in which the boy uses it. Also the needle's relationship to the length of the fingers might be an essential element.

ZAZZO:
We noticed during observations on children between seven and twelve in a cinema that during moments of excitement the boys had movements stretching towards the screen whereas the little girls had movements coming back towards their bodies: they touched their face or their chest. We took systematic photographs in ultra-violet light unknown to the children; on the parts of the film which were fairly exciting or which caused interest we had two very different attitudes for boys and girls apart, of course, from individual differences.

MEAD:
Dr. Zazzo showed me these pictures yesterday. This tendency of the girl to bring her hands back to the body is something we find in many societies. For example, in the balancing behaviour in the boy there seems to be more reaching-out, and if he balances with his own body he is likely to hold on to his penis, whereas the girl folds her arms or places them on to her head and shows more of a with-drawal into the self. This again might be dependent on a whole series of other factors but it does occur with quite remarkable

persistency. In a society like Bali where the men behave more like women in terms of extensor activities the men also touch their own bodies a good deal more and bring their hands back to their own body.

GREY WALTER:

Do you remember that delightful passage in *Huckleberry Finn* where Huck puts on a girl's dress to try and disguise himself and goes to visit a woman and is trying to get away with being a girl and she throws him something and instead of opening his legs to catch it as a girl would do, he closes them to catch it as a boy would do; I thought it was a most delightful scene.

MONNIER:

If we distinguish skilfulness in games and skilfulness in technical activities, we get the impression that here also the development in boys is somewhat different from that in girls. Boys may have the greatest skilfulness in games, but when they have to become trained in a technical professional activity, it takes a long time because skilfulness implies self-control. To become skilled, one must inhibit all kinds of impulsive gestures and effective expressions which are a hindrance to technical skilfulness. We have evidence that inhibition of these parasitic affective movements in technical training occurs somewhat later in boys than in girls.

MEAD:

There again we have to be sure whether this is because boys are reared by women and are developing a sort of counter-movement against the movement of their mother. Perhaps if a little boy could start imitating his father and working as his father works from the time he was very small, this sort of difference might disappear.

Now, to turn from this question of rhythms of work and types of work and types of climax structure to the question of creativity, which is a basic problem between men and women; there again, it is possible to make the simple historical point that in any society that has permitted women to do something as women they have become highly skilled. Most of the discussion that goes on today about the relative achievement of men and women is a discussion of the achievements of women in a man's field. We say, well, we have let women work with music now for hundreds of years and they do nothing; but actually we have only let them do something that has been perfected and elaborated by men, that is designated as male and which, therefore, may be expected to introduce a great many blocks and difficulties in the performance. We must consider the possibility that whenever a creative activity can be defined as female it may elicit the capacity in females; it will never be elicited as long as it is defined as male. I think that should always be systematically taken into account.

However, let us go on to a rather different point and that is the extent to which the male explores and works with the external world, and imposes form and structure on it, whereas the female tends to confine her activities more to her own body. This could be regarded as the basis of differences of creativity. Small girls, especially in as primitive society, are all well assured that if they wait they will have children; an individual woman may, of course, be unfortunate and not have a child, but the expected thing is that one will have a child and that one doesn't have to do anything whatsoever except *be*. If girls will continue simply to be girls until they are big enough, someone will marry them (in these primitive societies of which I speak every woman is married, at least once) and they will have children. Any urge towards any other form of creativity would be muted as compared with the possibility of making children, especially in a society where the production of children is so conspicuous because so few other things are produced that are of any importance. The climax structure and work rhythm come in again here also, I think, because the woman has a child, she doesn't have half a child, three-quarters of a child, or nine-tenths of a child, she has a child or she doesn't have a child. Now, in contrast to child-bearing, male tasks, in most parts of the world, can be quantitatively sub-divided— you build a house, and then you build a bigger house. Achievement can be graded, and compared, and you can go on from one achievement to another. Irreversibles in male achievement usually have to be phrased in biological terms similar to women's achievements— for example, that a man who has not begotten a son is not a man. But for most things, the difference between the single complete achievement, in a woman having one child or two children, and the graduated achievement of man who is continually going on to build new bridges, or to conquer new worlds in one form or another, seems to be a pretty systematic one.

At least in those societies that have been looked at we find this tendency for women to rest for a long period as small girls and at puberty and simply wait, not acquiring more than the minimum of skills that are necessary for marriage and then, having had children, to rest on their laurels and to feel this is an adequate enough achievement. This contrasts with the males' continually going on to more and more and more activity, and corresponds to the difference in

59

climax structure wherein male reproductive life may go on for a very long period with different degrees of continuity and discontinuity, whereas the female reproductive period is cut off sharply and clearly. These points, I think, must not be underestimated in their effect not only at the moment that they occur, but as expectations held out continuously to children.

LORENZ:

I am very much struck by the fact that when we speak of female creativity we are always thinking of a female's creativity in the man's field of work. Now how about the field of typical feminine activity in one culture—let us say weaving. I understand that in the early stages of our culture weaving was particularly feminine and the word 'wife' derived from 'weaving'. Is there any record whether the *technique* of weaving, the loom, was invented by a woman? I know of one instance of something which was definitely invented by women and by women exclusively, and that is the very intricate details and varieties of knitting, that is still being invented by women and I have seen my mother—all my anthropology is derived from observations of my own family—invent very intricate new patterns, but I don't see my mother inventing a loom.

MEAD:

I think that you could say that the women have invented the stitches. In ancient Peru, where we find every single stitch that has ever been thought of in weaving, weaving was done by women. But what you suggest is rather what I would expect also—that the women would invent stitches and the men would invent the loom.

HUXLEY:

On the other hand I understand that the Bayeux tapestry was not done by Queen Matilda's women at all, but by a guild of men embroiderers—the creativity there was in the hands of the men.

MEAD:

Yes, weaving in Peru was feminine and in Europe a great deal of it was masculine, but you get the same sort of invention in the stitch in both instances.

LORENZ:

I would like to know of cultures where the women do the fishing. Do you think or can you show there that the method of fishing is also invented by women, because that is what I expect, you see.

MEAD:

It is almost impossible to show how any of these methods were invented. Women have different methods from men, but that doesn't at all preclude the men having invented them for the women to use.

HUXLEY:

One very interesting changeover was that from boys to women in representing female parts on the stage. Once women were allowed to, they became great actresses. Does it mean that women are naturally better in interpretative roles than in creative ones?

MEAD:

It is possible the interpretative roles come easier. It is possible that all of those forms of creativity where a pattern is imposed on the material are more congenial to men and all of those forms where one responds to the form of material are more congenial to women. I would like to stress another point. Take for example mathematical ability: it may be that the most gifted mathematicians will always be men, that the real mathematical gift might occur in one-tenth of one per cent. of the male sex, but always in males. Then the maleness of mathematics gets defined from the genius. Or it may on the contrary simply be that a larger percentage of men than of women deal well with mathematics and the stereotype is set up and communicated to children that way. Or it may be that historically men have dealt with mathematics to such a degree that mathematics is thought of as male. I don't feel that any of our cultural material is of an order to do more than raise these questions.

FREMONT-SMITH:

Margaret, would you say that once a sex-differential role has been established, such as in reference to mathematics, that then it would be extremely easy for the society to perpetuate it, and rather difficult to break through and change it even though there wasn't any biological reason for it?

MEAD:

Yes, I would; furthermore if you take some of these very simple primitive people, they may count to 20 or 24. The brightest person in that group—a mathematical genius—might count up to 50 and might not be able to perpetuate it, whereas in the societies like ours people with relatively low IQ will learn algebra, because the whole society is permeated with mathematics.

HUXLEY:

Would you agree with the point which Konrad Lorenz raised yesterday, about a sex difference in readiness to be interested in and in ability to control mechanical devices? That is rather important in a mechanical society, and I should have thought as you change from the sort of crude mechanical technology of the 19th century to today's advanced technology of electronics and so on—from Lewis Mumford's paleotechnics to neotechnics—that would make a very considerable difference.

MEAD:

Except that, you see, electronic machinery is the sort of thing which is more congenial to a woman.

HUXLEY:

That is what I meant. The difference in mechanical ability would only be effective in the paleotechnic period.

ZAZZO:

Two remarks concerning this aptitude for mathematics which is supposed to be greater among boys than among girls. I think there are two factors—a factor of spatial organization which seems to be more developed, more precocious, among small boys than among small girls, and an affective factor. We might have some doubt as regards a real difference in aptitude for mathematics between the sexes; it is less a question of aptitude than of the relations which may exist between affectivity and logical thought. We can show that even if boys succeed on an average better than girls, nevertheless 90 per cent. of our schoolboys fail to understand mathematics, and this failure is not due, I think, to a lack of aptitude for mathematics. A person of average intelligence can go quite far in the realm of mathematics if he is not hindered by all kinds of affective difficulties. There must be a reduction in affective reactions if logical thought is to proceed harmoniously and clearly. This reduction perhaps works less well for girls on an average than for boys.

HUXLEY:

I think Dr. Zazzo has made a very important point—that you are dealing with something which is not a specific aptitude to perform some action, but what in biology we call a pre-adaptation or a prerequisite for such performance. These prerequisites may differ considerably and may have a very big effect on final results.

If we compare two groups of boys and of girls of the same age we do not in fact observe any significant difference in the development of logical functions. On the other hand we note slight differences in the formation of spatial representation, for example when it is a question of transformations and developments of geometric solids. Moreover, we note that these differences, which are very little pronounced among young children, take on greater importance with age. But sexual differences are not the only factors involved, there are also factors of exercise and, because of this, of school and cultural environment. Those children who at all ages have much richer possibilities of manipulation and visual-tactile exploration have as a general rule better spatial representation. The mental image in its spatial form seems originally to be the interiorization of movements of exploration (Piaget & Inhelder, 1948). This is why we think that the differences observed between the performances of boys and girls are not only linked to sex but are due rather to the intervention of a number of causes, among others, sensori-motor exercise and the school and cultural 'climate.'

DE SAUSSURE :
I would like to make a remark along the same lines as that made by Professor Zazzo. In the clinic we see from time to time women who protest against their femininity, accepting masculine activities and showing even great aptitude for mathematics and for mechanical questions, simply because their affectivity is directed to this side. The question I should like to ask is this : in certain primitive societies, does one see enough women with such a desire, so that all of a sudden an activity which had been masculine up to then is thereafter taken up by women?

MEAD :
I have never seen a primitive society where one had a very highly developed masculine protest in women. I have seen societies where women have played a great many roles that in other societies were masculine—where they fought, climbed coconut trees, took long voyages and things of that sort and did them as well as, or in some cases to the exclusion of men, but the particular kind of release of energy that we see in our society in a woman who wants to be masculine and wants to show what she can do, and that she can compete, I think is a more sophisticated development. We don't have really any true analogues at the primitive level. For instance, the Eskimo woman knows how to build a house as well as an Eskimo man does,

and very often she is stuck and has to build a house. She may be travelling on one sled with two children, and her husband on another sled with the other and doesn't get there. As she builds the house she comments: 'This is not of course a real house, this is just a put-together shack of no importance, that a mere woman is cutting out of snow. This amounts to nothing àt all. This is not a house, it is just a shelter against the elements'. I think that position is a little more common in primitive societies than the other one.

GREY WALTER:
Could you tell us something about the aspect of personality which is reflected in our Western culture in hobbies, which often reflect rather more faithfully the personality of an individual than his occupation does? It is rather rare in English society for a woman to have a hobby, but I gather in America there are women's clubs and so on that fill the place of hobbies in men's lives.

MEAD:
Well, my first general statement would be that hobbies are male. You may have derivative hobbies in the female. If all the little boys that a little girl knows collect stamps, she may collect a few.

HUXLEY:
Is this so in primitive cultures too?

MEAD:
It is so in any society that I know anything about. Sheer hobbies in the sense that one has them in England don't exist in primitive societies, they are a special rather late development. But the elaboration of leisure in theatricals, in offerings, and so forth, tends to be a male activity in all the societies that we know anything about. One of the things that happens is that the minute you get an elaboration of leisure you get this preoccupation of men with activities that superficially look feminine—dressing dolls, cutting out pretty little cut-out things, cutting leaves and flowers up. In Bali the men spend hours and hours cutting pig fat into roses, and then some more hours fashioning little pigs out of rose leaves. An enormous amount of time goes into these activities, almost as if when a society gets to a point when it has leeway for leisure then it is possible for males as bi-sexual creatures to play games at what it would be like to be a woman. I think this generalization could be supported, for example, in relation to the arts, and the tendency at many periods for the arts to be regarded as feminine. That is, you

64

have first a period of extreme rigour, like the American frontier, and no art at all. Then as the arts develop more and more, they are first taken up by women and then they are taken over by men. Most of these symbolic activities, hobbies—stamp collecting, gardening, fishing—may be in this class. Consider the efforts that a culture has to go to make a woman fish for pleasure. However, I know two or three women executives now who fish.

LORENZ:

Oh, but in Florida nowadays sport fishing is nearly an exclusively feminine occupation.

MEAD:

But they are not fishing for pleasure!

GREY WALTER:

The modern Atlantic woman has two lives, in a way. I mean that her longevity is great, so she has a pre-menopausal and post-menopausal life, and she isn't usually greatly encumbered with children in the second life. In your experience of developing American culture are women of post-menopausal age becoming hobby-ridden?

MEAD:

No. They are becoming social-organization-ridden. Clubs, community services, good deeds—a proliferation of inter-personal relations. But painting, for example, is work again. You see, painting is done in response to the belief that one *ought* to find out how to express one's personality, and I don't think should be properly defined as leisure.

If you look the world over, the participation of women in games is extraordinarily small. There is one small case-history (Wolfenstein, 1946, Mead, 1955) in this particular field. About ten years ago, a group of us conceived the idea of short-circuiting the relationship between contemporary child psychology and the child reader. The idea was to get psychoanalysts and anthropologists and child developers to plan what four-year-olds ought to read and then get a book written and give it to them. We went about this in a very elaborate way, we convened a group of specialists and the specialists enumerated what a little girl should know about having a little sibling, that mother would get tired, there was no room on mother's lap, and things of that sort, and that she should be allowed to help with the baby clothes. But the male writer who wrote the story invented a creature called a *rampatan*, and, while mother and father had a baby, little Sally had a *rampatan*. And a *rampatan* could be anything you liked. It could fly, it could swim, it could go on the land. It could have the head of a rabbit and the tail of a snake, or the head of a lion and the body of a pussycat. It was a delightful story and after it was written, we tried it out on mothers, on children and on fathers. The children knew what the *rampatan* was about. The fathers knew what the *rampatan* was about, but the women said that they couldn't see what in the world this *rampatan* had to do with a woman having a baby.

GREY WALTER:

I want to get my picture clear of how you are looking at our present culture. Do you yourself notice, or has there been described, a significant sex difference in the attitude of children to the non-reflexive diversions such as television?

MEAD:

No, I should say not. In the United States at present, so far as I know, there is no difference in the spectatorship of girls and boys in spite of the fact that the content is on the whole masculine. Now whether that means anything except that parents use the television set as a baby sitter, and whether we are talking about children or whether we are talking about adults, I wouldn't be sure. But of course spectator sports in adults depend on men far more than women.

FREMONT-SMITH

There is one point that I would like to bring up here. In human societies there is the greatest possible difficulty in separating out biological sex differences from the influence of the social organization. I want to come back to Konrad's remark yesterday about the bull playing with the little male bulls and ask whether we haven't made a false dichotomy between the human race and the lower biological species, in the assumption that in animals we can see quite easily the pure impact of genetically determined sex, whereas in humans we have to disentangle it from the culture. I wonder whether it may not be true in a good many animals that the culture plays a role right from the beginning also?

HUXLEY:

But there isn't any culture in animals!

LORENZ:
Practically none is known. There is a certain cultural element in social, sexual and nest-building behaviour in chimps, as Hayes (1951) and Nissen very clearly showed. Tradition is important to such an extent that it is difficult to breed chimps if you haven't got a sexually experienced one, and you have got to start with one wild-caught chimp in a colony in order to teach them how to copulate. And then hand-reared chimps don't nest-build, though the motor patterns involved are very probably instinctive activities. But wild-caught ones do build a nest, and there was hitherto only one captivity-reared chimp on record who knew how to do it, and he was reared by a wild-caught mother. And that is practically all I know about animal culture!

FREMONT-SMITH:
What about bulls?

LORENZ:
All that is purely innate.

HUXLEY:
Culture, surely, is only definable as the result of the cumulative transmission of experience.

LORENZ:
Julian Huxley once said that the traditional knowledge of dangerous predators which I have demonstrated in the jackdaw was hitherto the only example of this kind, but since then Nissen and Hayes have found two or three other instances.
But I want to ask something which is pertinent to this question. Vertebrates in general are protogynous hermaphrodites, which in simple words means that they are hermaphroditic in the general layout of their anatomy and that, as a rule, female characters develop before male characters. For example, many young birds are hen-coloured and develop cock plumage later on. There are very few exceptions to this rule. There was one paper by a man named Winterbottom (1929) which Julian lent me and made me read about 20 years ago, and this man made the difference between aretic and aphroditic characters in species. Aretic characters are characters developed in phylogeny by the male sex first and aphroditic characters are characters developed by the female sex first. For instance nipples, the utriculus prostaticus and other primarily female characters which men carry are aphroditic characters. All of you know that

67

the distribution of pubic hair when it first grows is female, that mammary glands grow for a certain time in the pubescent male and so on, and therefore, I always took as a matter of course that little boys wore skirts, when I was young, and generally are treated as girls and look like girls. And in Holland there are regions where the little boys up to five years are dressed absolutely as girls. In the islands of Vollendam and Markendam as the only sex-distinguishing mark they have a round disk sewn to their bonnets to tell whether they are male or female. I was very much surprised when I heard about this society where all children were dressed and treated as boys, and my question is now how is the little boy in our society discouraged from behaving like Ma? What are the reinforcements for imitating Pa and not Ma? And, vice versa, how are the reverse reinforcements effected in that New Guinea society, and do the little boys in this society retain some feminine characters afterwards?

MEAD:

I should say that in our society a baby boy is discouraged from behaving like a female from the moment he is born. The first time his mother picks him up in her hands, her hands are saying to him 'You are a little male'. A great proportion of his learning is communicated kinaesthetically very, very young. In all the societies we have been talking about it is the mother who is the operative person. But in Manus the father is exceedingly important, and has become steadily more important in handling little girls, and I think this case more or less supports the position I have been taking all along, that it is the mother who makes the child into otherness, if it is a boy. American mothers call their children Caxton and Jones and Smith now at the age of two—'Go wash your face, Jones', they say with a heavy voice that is going to turn these little boys into proper males. The goading of males into being males that goes on in the hands of women, and the treating them as 'other', as 'different', as 'not myself', is very great. But just let men raise the little girls—they try to make girls just like themselves. The tendency of fathers who rear daughters to turn them into males and want them to behave like males, and to move like males, and show the attitudes of males, is probably stronger than the tendency in the mother towards the little Lord Fauntleroy, wishing her son had been a girl. But the mother who makes her little boy feminine differs from the father, who says, 'This is the way to behave—stand like *this*, hold your punt like *this*, paddle like *this*, don't paddle like that, paddle like this'. He is not saying 'I wish you were a boy', he is saying 'behave like a human being, there is only one way to behave'.

Dr. Sears (1953) has done a study of male and female choices in nursery school-children, and the extent to which the girl will want to do the thing the father does, and be encouraged to do it, while the boy is discouraged by the mother from wanting to do the things that she does.

LORENZ:
But I am still astonished that the boy treated by his mother in that way does not become a female-imitation man, but becomes a real man. He is taught not to be like a female, but why does he imitate his father—which he does.

MEAD:
There are many societies in which the small male has almost no contact with the father at all, and where the mother has to do the teaching, so we have societies in which the mother teaches the boy to be a male-like creature, and we have societies in which the mother teaches the boy to be a female-like creature.

LORENZ:
Well, I had better come out and be honest about what I am aiming at. I do believe that there is a certain unlearned element—something like an IRM—which makes the little boy actually seek for somebody to take over the father role. Sylvia Klimpfinger has evidence for that in a hospital—a hostel—where all the children are reared by the female staff alone, and all these children—the boys more significantly than the girls—go for the gardener who is the only male accessible to them. This led me to suspect that there might be an unlearned preference for what to imitate—boys to imitate Pa and for girls to imitate Ma.

MEAD:
Well, I suspect that there is a very early capacity for sex-differentiation, and that there may well be an IRM by which female babies discriminate between male and female nurses. You would not necessarily have to say the child was seeking for a model, but with the capacity to discriminate and then with the developing of the sense of the self, the search for the particular type of model may begin.

BUCKLE:
As to why the boy tends to imitate the male, surely we must consider why the boy rejects the female. I doubt whether it is a

69

sufficient condition that the mother expects the child to be not like her. Surely there is a rejection of the mother by the child.

MEAD:

Ultimately, in adult life we have the rejection. But is there a mechanism in the young child that, for instance, rejects the female? Dr. Arthur Mirsky (unpublished research) did a study of the sense of smell in boys and girls, taking into account Freud's statement that we paid for our upright posture with giving up our sense of smell. He found that up to puberty boys' and girls' sense of smell was identical, and from puberty until middle age men's sense of smell goes way down, and in late middle age it is restored and is again quite comparable to the female. That would look to me like a clear case of a mechanism of non-identification with the mother, that the girl has to keep her identification with the smell of a female, has to accept milk and the smell of milk, and the whole female body odour. One of the things that the male does is to reject the smell connected with maternity and infancy. This happens at puberty and not in early childhood.

BUCKLE:

There is a good deal of fantasy evidence, isn't there, that might be produced here—the male fantasy of the fear of the women, the dentate vagina, the Island of Amazons, and so on. As you said yesterday, these are all characteristically male fantasies which form part of a whole complicated defence against a fear of women. This may go back and be connected in some way to the original situation of care.

MEAD:

And vice versa. You also first get rejection fantasies in the female. The only question would be whether with the parent of the same sex the fantasies are comparable because the girl, in rejecting or being fascinated by the stranger—the father who only comes home at night —is in a different position from the boy who has to cope with something that is there all day long, every day, every minute.

ERIKSON:

Maybe for later discussion it would be important to differentiate between various forms of rejection. One can speak of fear of women on the part of the boys in the sense that they have fantasies as to what might happen to themselves if they *do* something *to* women —that is one thing. The other rejection would be based on an identification with women—how would it feel to *be* a woman in spite of otherness in body structure. There is also the fear of pregnancy aggravated by such questions as to where and how will the baby come out, and what it would do to a boy's body.

A second point I wanted to make for future discussion is that the example given by Dr. Lorenz can probably be broken down into any number of part mechanisms. You said there may be an intrinsic search for a father in boys. In your example the gardener was the only available man. But where there is some choice, it may well be that the gardener would still be preferred. He is a man who works outside, who does something to the ground, has tools, has a technique. I would think a clerk sitting in an office in the same building would not have attracted quite the same attention. In other words locomotion could be important, the outdoorness, the handling of tools, the circumscribed technique—all of these things.

MEAD:

We have been able to watch the identification formed by several small boys whose fathers are intellectuals in households that share a Peruvian cleaning man who works with a vacuum cleaner—the little boys adore the Peruvian cleaning man with the vacuum cleaner.

RÉMOND:

I should like to ask Margaret Mead what, according to her, are the attributes of masculinity. Don't you think that 'authority' might be one of the attributes of the masculine sex, which is found in many present societies and perhaps even in primitive societies? Authority would go with initiative, while on the feminine side one would find rather submission and passiveness. All this could be attached to the one of the two persons who went in search of the other sex. It is the man who makes the approach to the woman, rather than the contrary, which gives him a certain initiative and finally a certain authority which imposes his presence on the other. From this there would follow a whole series of other qualities which would be masculine qualities. What do you think then of the importance of this division of authority between the two sexes?

MEAD:

I would like to break that into two, I think: the related authority of father or mother—that is, which parent, the father or the mother, is the more appropriate disciplining person—which is one part of the picture which builds up into a husband-wife relationship, and the other point about the male seeking the female. Now among my head-hunters in New Guinea, the Iatmul and Mundugumor, the female seeks the male, and the males say it would be much too dangerous to make a proposal to a woman unless you knew whether she wanted you or not. So that all the provocative initiative comes from the women and the women send insults to the men, which arouses the men's sense of initiative and, shall we say, authority, to a sufficient point so that the men are then able to court the women. I think it is both a fairly complicated problem and also a very simple one on an anatomical basis. It looks reasonably clear that the physical initiative belongs to the male, and passivity, and receptivity and intraception belongs to the female, and any extreme reversal of this position is likely to be awkward and inconvenient. Nevertheless, there are so many stages and phases and repeats and elaborations in this whole picture that it is possible to turn the female into a provocative, seeking, teasing person.

ERIKSON:
I think we should add these two words 'awkward' and 'inconvenient' to the one 'expensive' which I suggested earlier for inclusion in our special vocabulary.

INTERVAL

MEAD:
I think perhaps the next thing we ought to tackle is the implicaations for sex differences of the very protracted human infancy and the question of what we are able to say at present about the stages that the psychoanalyst usually calls pre-genital. This is the point where Erik Erikson and I overlap greatly, for I have relied a great deal through the last 20 years on his clinical work and his charts of pre-genital development. As he built them up, I have tried to apply that to different cultures and having done so to emerge with new hyotheses that we could test. The first point I want to raise is the question of *latency*, because it seems to me that this is a problem where we again overlap with the animal world. To what extent the young child of each sex, after a period of fairly vivid affective relationship to parents and to its own body has a sort of—I don't know whether I should use the word 'moratorium', because you are using it for your adolescent period, Erik, but in a sense it is a kind of moratorium.

72

ERIKSON:
A psychosexual moratorium: the later one I would call psycho-social.

MEAD:
A psychosexual moratorium then—a period when what looks like a straight line of sexual development is held in abeyance and the child turns away from the affective libidinized relationships to other people and concentrates on its own learning. One of the very interesting points has been whether there was such a thing as latency in girls. We have pretty good evidence for most societies that there is a short period for boys. It may sometimes be rather artificially defined; for instance, if children are sent to school at six, latency begins at six if it hasn't begun before. The child is taken away and subjected to an education outside the home, which in practically all instances is mediated by a stranger in some shape or other. There is indeed, an almost universal use in human societies of the stranger as the educative influence to break with the home, whether through an initiation ceremony or in school (Hart, 1955). In girls it is a very open question as to whether there is this withdrawal from psycho-sexual activity to anything like the same extent as in boys. In any society where girls continue to be treated as desirable little feminine objects you get a consistent and uninterrupted line of giggling self-conscious behaviour, with the girls giving a clear picture of being more or less available for sexual advances at any point as far as they themselves are concerned (with, of course, a large number of social restrictions built up around them). Fright or fear may be built over this receptivity, extreme shyness may be laid over it. But there is a contrasting picture between boys and girls as if this period of latency functions some way for the boy in a way it doesn't for the girls.
We have had relatively little information about the psychosexual development of the girl as compared with the boy. Psychoanalysis was built up on assumptions about boys and assumptions about the way little girls felt about little boys, and most women who have done any psychoanalytic work on childhood have suffered from a masculine protest which is a little more extreme than the typical one, so a lot of psychoanalytic literature on girls has been concerned with revolt of one kind or another against Freudian theory that in many cases is utterly unrelated to girls. But by one of those extraordinary, happy accidents, two weeks ago I was sent a paper by an American child-analyst named Dr. Judith Kestenberg (in press) and was very much struck with it.
Dr. Kestenberg is working with a slightly different approach to the

73

whole problem of the hymen from any approach that I know of. I have tended, on the whole, to see the function of the hymen as protecting the juvenile male; it does not, after all, protect the juvenile female against any full-grown male; it may be a protection if you build up an elaborate ritual and send men to jail if they have sex relations with too young a child, but the hymen itself does not present any particular barrier to a full-grown male. It does, however, present a certain degree of discouragement in adolescent play, so that one of the possible ways in which the hymen may have functioned is to decrease the amount of adolescent and pre-adolescent sex play and to prolong the period of play without penetration, which occurs in so many peasant societies where you have the type of sex relations called 'bundling', in which the pair of future lovers will spend nights with each other but without puncturing the hymen. A good proportion of this looked as if it were a way of deferring sex activities for males. Now Dr. Kestenberg is advancing a quite different theory, based on very extensive work with little girls: that the hymen's function is to make the female genital inaccessible to complete exploration (see Birch, 1954).

We have a great deal of clinical material to suggest a failure on the part of the young female completely to integrate any picture of the inside of her body. Dr. Kestenberg suggests that what the hymen does is to interfere with the female child's self-exploration and that this defective exploration combined with a vaginal sensation which she cannot localize are important elements in the development of early female sexuality. The unrealized, or only partially realized, interior of the vagina becomes projected on dolls, on puppies, on parts of the mother's body, on all the small round, soft, pleasant objects that the little girl carries around and cherishes. There is no doubt that we do have a greater acceptance of such objects on the part of girls than of boys. You can get boys to play with dolls and, by a considerable amount of effort, you can equalize the playing time between them and girls for a short period. But there seems to be a rather constant acceptance, on the part of girls, of dolls and doll-substitutes. Dolls are not universal in primitive societies, but they are universal in high civilization, which suggests possibly that one of the necessary prerequisites to psychosexual maturity in the female of the sort that will fit into a high civilization may be this period of delay and the long practice at mothering. Dr. Kestenberg's is a very new hypothesis and is based almost entirely on clinical material. We haven't had time to check it across the cultures that I know something about. There are some other bits of it that are very interesting. She discusses the tendency of the girl to nag and identifies

74

very carefully several periods in the girl's development when she nags. The nagging of women is notorious in many cultures; the mother nagging the child is an exceedingly widespread phenomenon. Dr. Kestenberg suggests that this nagging which can be identified in the behaviour of little girls, is the response to unlocalized vaginal sensations that may begin very early and are unplaced but irritating.

TANNER:

I just want to put a question to Lorenz. Do other primates have hymens or not?

LORENZ:

I don't know.

MEAD:

Guinea-pigs?

TANNER:

That is different. In guinea-pigs and in other rodents there is a vaginal plug which disappears as a result of oestrogen secretion. The disappearance is one of the signs of puberty in these animals. But oestrogen doesn't do anything to the human hymen—I mean directly!

MEAD:

As far as I have been able to find out, no one who is an authority on primate anatomy knows of any primate that has a hymen. This is distinctively a human characteristic. Whether this particular theoretical formulation of Kestenberg's is anything more than suggestive I am not prepared to say at this stage, but I do think that one of our problems in the differentiation of male and female is the type of early sexuality (Henry, 1941) and the type of early maternity that are experienced by the girl. One finds that girl children as compared with boys are more prone to put things inside things and those things in turn inside something else. Erik Erikson is going to show us presently slides of contrasting play constructions of girls and boys.

Certainly something that needs very careful exploration is the precursor of later sexual behaviour in little boys and girls. Here again, we have a terrific degree of contrast. There are societies that forbid all childish manipulation of the genitals; there are societies in which adults put children to sleep playing with their genitals, and there are societies in which groups of people are more or less joined together by genital association. Among very simple Indians, like the Kaingang in South America, where there is a sort of marriage linkage group—a man will sleep with this or that woman for a fairly short period and children will be added to groups by a very conscious and elaborate sexual manipulation quite young. So one has all varieties of behaviour, from adults who participate in the capacity of young infants to be aroused to societies in which there is a very sharp taboo on any such arousal. I think this is necessary to say because there have been theories that the taboo on masturbation was a necessary concomitant of humanity and that is simply not so, if we follow the range across different sorts of societies. I think I mentioned last year the Siriono and Lepchas where the boys of twelve have access to their older brothers' wives, and where all sexual competition is removed very young. They have as sex partners, the wives of those who would normally be prohibitive, frightening, competitive, towards themselves. Both Siriono and Lepchas are people who, in spite of several hundred years' exposure to higher civilization, have been remarkably resistant to its influence.

There is also a considerable amount of material from complex societies which shows that, for the élite classes, there is a tendency to postpone sexuality for a longer period than in, say, a peasant group or a working-class group in a large city. The point to which the society permits, indulges and enjoys the potential sexuality of young children, and the way in which that is made part of the social organization is another factor which we have to think about in this sex differentiation question. I would think, Konrad, that we ought to have some cross-referencing from animals and birds to human beings about the way the sense of the one body and the sense of the other are developed. Case histories of individuals show that never having seen another human body can be important in determining the psychosexual development and can be considered with the sorts of experience that a child has with its own body and with the bodies of its parents.

LORENZ:
I think self-exploration of that type, curiosity of one's own body, is something very specifically human—the difference between the highest anthropoids and humans may be only quantitative, but if so it is huge.

ERIKSON:
By human, do you mean the species or the culture?

76

LORENZ:

The species. I am sure that this interest in one's own body, self-exploration, and so on, is the same practically for all human beings.

GREY WALTER:

The mirror test would be pretty specific for that, wouldn't it? There are very few animals below man that take any interest in their own reflection.

LORENZ:

Yes, certainly. The mirror deceives the animal into thinking there is another animal. He is deceived, but still he is interested, he grabs behind the mirror.

GREY WALTER:

But there is no identification.

LORENZ:

No, there is no identification, they do not realize that it is them.

GREY WALTER:

Chimpanzees do, I think.

LORENZ:

Well, I don't know—I think they would.

GREY WALTER:

I seem to remember Lashley told me they act as if they do.

HUXLEY:

It would be very difficult for birds, for instance, to build up a body image because so many of their reactions are to specific releasers. For instance, parent song-birds react equally well to an artificial gape— provided that it is coloured right and has an artificial tongue in it —as they do to their own young. They don't react to their young, they react to a coloured pattern which wobbles. In the same way the male robin reacts aggressively, not to a rival bird, but to a patch of red feathers. It is not a question of a body image, but of an automatic releaser.

LORENZ:

Yes, and actually the treatment of their own body shows you very prettily how little self-exploration takes place in birds. Delacour's observation (personal communication) of the Mandarin drake shows that, too: you will remember the bird which failed to grow the ornamental fan feather and yet persisted for years preening the empty air above its back where its feather ought to have been.

HUXLEY:
He just reacted automatically, like the song-bird parent who puts food into the artificial mouth.

ERIKSON:
Concerning the question of latency, if one takes the whole life-span of any animal and compares it with the human life-span, is the possibility of genital intercourse as delayed in any animal species as it is in the human being?

FREMONT-SMITH:
In a condensed life-span you might miss the latency because it would take place in a few days, or weeks, instead of several years.

HUXLEY:
An elephant lives absolutely a long time but he becomes mature relatively early compared to a man. Man is undoubtedly partially neotenous or paedomorphic, in that his juvenile stage has been relatively prolonged. Indeed, sometimes it is prolonged into the sexually adult phase. You don't get any brow ridges in adult human males, because their absence in all primate young has in him been prolonged into adult life.

LORENZ:
And my argument would be that this retardation of becoming a real adult also implies a long residence in the phase of exploratory curiosity which in animals is extremely limited and in all of us, in humans, persists.

TANNER:
Nevertheless, the primate growth curve is very much closer to that of man than it is to that of any of the other mammals. The dichotomy that one sees in comparing mammalian growth curves is between rhesus and chimpanzee and man on the one hand and the others on the other (see Tanner, 1955). If the psychological inference you draw from this is correct it would be very interesting to know what goes on in the rhesus' and the chimp's minds during this time.

HUXLEY:

If I recollect right, a chimp becomes sexually mature at about seven or eight years and may live to forty or fifty. I should have thought, in reference to what Konrad has said about exploratory curiosity being prolonged in primates and especially in man, that this is a biological necessity. If you are going to become a successful biological type through the possession of greater intelligence, you want a longer time for learning.

LORENZ:

It is one of the many conditions that made man Man.

HUXLEY:

And as J. B. S. Haldane pointed out years ago, a pre-condition of that was arboreal life with only one young at a time: otherwise you would have competition *in utero* between the foetuses, with the death of the slower growing ones. So there would have been automatic selection favouring rapid development *in utero*, and the effect of this would have been carried over into post-natal life. It is one of the most beautiful insights that Haldane ever had.

MEAD:

There is a good deal of evidence (Mead, 1935, passim) that this period of latency and exploratory curiosity in boys is stronger than in girls, although I have seen one society where it was reversed, but reversed expensively. This was among the Tchambuli, which was the one group that I worked with where there was a very striking reversal of the expected personality characteristics of each sex: it was not a matrilineal society with structural reversal, but just personality reversal. The men were gossipy, giggly, catty, they went shopping, they spent all their time on their clothes, they had given up warfare and although they were head-hunting people they bought their victims, and then one person held the head-hunting victim while a little boy went and stuck a spear into him and then he was a big man. The women, on the other hand, were bold, brusque, adequate. They were co-operative, they worked in groups, they had moveable stoves so that whenever a group of women wanted to do anything each one carried her own stove and set it down next to the other one, so that there were twenty women cooking and slapping each other on the back. The women did all the marketing and were responsible for the productivity of the society. The men were the consumers. The women had shaved heads and the men wore ringlets, and if they didn't have ringlets, they made ringlets. So that it was a

79

quite striking reversal on the general personality level. Now usually in societies that have initiation, the common male initiation is in a group, and the common female initiation is for a single little girl when she reaches menarche. It is very difficult to get enough little girls at menarche at the same moment, so if you are going to pay attention to the biological reality you have to take one girl at a time. But the Tchambuli had reversed this and they initiated one little boy at a time and fussed over him and dressed him. He acted like a shy little debutante. In this group the little girls were very much like little boys, active, enterprising, curious. It was the little girl who went everywhere I went, carried my camera and wanted to know how the camera worked, and showed the characteristics that we associate with small boys. So the greater curiosity of boys is certainly reversible, but reversible under rather extreme conditions.

It is interesting to speculate whether the post-menopausal stage in women in which women are freed from child-bearing is a stage of the same sort as the prolonged childhood that gives males a period of freedom from psychosexual preoccupation. If women have survived through the menopause they then usually have a higher expectation of life than the men. In many societies post-menopausal women play an exceedingly important role as the custodians of the past, the responsible element of conservation in the society. This may again represent a biological change, because the menopause is also something that does not occur among primates—or at least it is not a regular aspect of primate physiology as we know it at present.

LORENZ:

The oldest chimp of known age, who is 34, Alpha, has had a baby this year. Only a few years ago chimps were still supposed to be perfectly sterile and perfectly senile at this age.

But do you know what Fraser-Darling the stagman wrote on the subject: he said the more tradition, culture, intelligence, personal learning play a role in the ecology of animals, the more important, and valuable, were the old individuals, even if they did not reproduce any more. This, of course, is the case with deer; where the old, old females which are years past reproduction are the leaders and the most powerful social agents; everybody obeys these old, very old ladies. Fraser-Darling's principle might apply to man more than to other living creatures, particularly as compared with anthropoids.

MEAD:

I think in primate societies the old males are treated very badly and have very low social duties.

80

LORENZ:

Well, I think that's again dependent on something different. The old male is simply chased out by the usurper of his dominant position —that happens with baboons in zoos.

MEAD:

Yes, but this type of dominance is not based on the same sort of knowledge that the old deer has.

ZAZZO:

I should like to come back to this definition of the period of latency. I don't want to minimize the psychosexual reactions in defining this period, but I wonder whether there isn't a certain danger in using these psychosexual reactions as a starting point, as an essential explanatory basis for the definition of this period from six to ten-eleven years. It seems to me that there is a much more general phenomenon of which the sexual reactions are only a factor. It is the general reactions of sociability and of affectivity which are obviously different at that age from what they were previously.

This period of latency is not a radical break with what went before. One notes that even in children between three and six years there are important differences in the social reactions of boys and girls, the boys' reactions being much less affective than the girls'. In the kindergarten, girls are often together, they have activities involving two or three; the boys are much more isolated in their games and other activities. It seems to me that this is accentuated during the period of latency. The contrast that I would like to point out also is that between the affective reactions of the period of three-six years and the social behaviour, the collective life, which starts from six-seven years onwards. Now this form of sociableness is very different from what can be observed previously, and even if there are sexual components there are also others of an intellectual nature. From six-seven years it seems that boys and girls have many more objective interests and activities of a logical, intellectual kind leading to a social life with children of their own age, and to the formation of groups of the same age, which was not the case before six-seven years. This activity continues up to eleven-twelve years; at twelve years it splits up again and one sees again the formation of pairs of friends. Before that there is a reaction of the social group, of the school group, against pairs of friends. One of my colleagues at the Sorbonne, Mr. Cousinet, noted that during the school period between seven and twelve years the whole group reacts

F   81

aggressively against the formation of pairs. I think, then, that there is a danger in relating the whole description of the period of latency to purely sexual behaviour, the word 'latency' being itself dangerous. We observe a much wider affective phenomenon of which sexuality is only one aspect.

MEAD:

Well, in using the term 'latency' I am perfectly prepared simply to define this phase as a phase when the child gives up overt competition with adults and goes in for a long period of sociability with peers while it is learning. The thing that it seems one finds almost everywhere is the boys giving up the close relationship to the family and going off by themselves. There are societies where the children are kept very warmly and closely in the family and the group does not live in large villages and you may not find children's groups, but whenever there is a large village where there are enough children to play together, then the tendency to play together in a group seems to develop. Here again we have the problem as to whether one thinks of man as having originally lived in towns of two or three hundreds—because if you take a group of semi-nomadic mountain people, such as one finds in parts of New Guinea, there isn't any group of children to play with. There will be the rare family that has three little boys, and they may have a much better time than other people, but children's gangs simply don't exist. I think we have to consider the gang, or the peer group, as a potentiality, but we can't include it as a necessary condition of maturation because living conditions often wouldn't make it possible. A children's play group where children meet for two days once a year is a very different sort of experience from playing together for half of every day.

In using the term psychosexual, I was not referring it only to sexuality but to the difference between the period when the little boy will still treat his father as a rival and the period when he more or less gives that up and consents to wait and roam, and acquire a fair number of skills before he comes back into the rivalry position with adult males. We do have very striking contrasts here between the rivalry of tiny children and that of ten-year-olds. Again culture can accentuate this difference. Among the Mundugumor, little boys of seven will stand up and defy their father over the sister because the sister is supposed to be the proper exchange for a brother's wife. But the males among the Mundugumor are always taking their daughters and exchanging them for extra wives for themselves. And so these small boys of six and seven years old stand up and defy their fathers in a row over a woman, when the sister is considerably older than they are. Such an extreme precocity, in terms of size and ability, is certainly a distortion of what one might normally expect.

MONNIER:

Sending the child to school at the age of six is more than an artificial social intervention in its development. From an electro-physiological standpoint, I think we would all agree that between five and seven there are definite signs in the EEG which point to the fact that the brain of the child has acquired adaptive functions. Because of this maturation of the brain and new adaptive functions, the child is now able to proceed from the exploration of his body to the exploration of the social surroundings, including the school collectivity. Young Arabs I had the opportunity to observe in Beirut, where there is no school obligation, develop spontaneously at this age of six to seven a definite social activity, in spite of the lack of school training. They start to sell things on the street and develop a kind of productive activity.

MEAD:

You can get this change much earlier. For instance, among the Aymara of Peru, four-year-olds are sent out as herders of whole herds of little pigs. Groups of them go out together and they will work together in a way that you don't normally expect to see until children are six or seven. Among the Manus play groups are formed between two and three: and play groups of the same general type that Professor Zazzo was describing as so very characteristic of a later stage.

GREY WALTER:

In regard to the electrophysiological correlates of development and latency I think one should add that, at any rate in our culture, the scatter of this second climacteric in children's brainwaves is very much wider than six to seven years; in fact, the thing that astonishes nearly everyone who studies this subject is the enormously wide scatter of the date at which children are through their second EEG climacteric, which is centred roughly around the school-entry age, about five or six. At that age there is a very wide distribution of degrees of cerebral maturity.

MEAD:

How about sex differences?

83

GREY WALTER:
As far as we can see—we have made quite careful analyses statistically—none of this scatter relates to sex differences at all; the distribution curves for little boys and girls superimpose quite exactly.

DE SAUSSURE:
I just wanted to recall that among the characteristics of the period of latency Freud stressed the appearance of defence mechanisms. I think that these defence mechanisms play an important part also in the differentiation between the sexes because, particularly for boys, they are partly a defence against affectivity and partly an intellectualization. With this intellectualization there is an isolation between feeling and the intellect which is probably much better developed in the boy than in the girl. The latter can maintain feelings much longer, or if she protests she does it rather by means of an hysterical repression whereas the boy's way would be rather through obsessional defence mechanisms.

HUXLEY:
There are two or three points to consider. One is the point that has already been brought up with regard to the slowing of development and the prolongation of infancy. Konrad Lorenz was telling me yesterday how very intelligent dolphins and porpoises appear to be; I don't know whether we know anything about their rate of development, but that of whales is incredibly fast. A whale which will weigh 100 tons when adult weighs several tons at birth after only about eleven months' gestation; it becomes sexually mature at two or three, and dies of old age, as far as we know, before twenty. It would be very interesting to know whether the development of dolphins is similar.

Another quite different but very interesting point: my wife reminded me that in the Museum at Tréguier in Brittany there is a remarkable exhibit—the plaits of hair of Renan, the great writer and theologian, which were cut off at the age of nine. In those days little Breton boys, I don't know whether of all classes, were brought up with long hair and dressed as girls in order that the fairies shouldn't steal them. It is perhaps of some further interest that Renan was very much dominated by his sister Henriette. I also remember seeing recently a photograph of Oscar Wilde in boyhood: his mother dressed him as a little girl—a fact which again may be significant for his future development.

Finally, in one tribe, I think it is the Bons they are called, in Orissa in India, the women are very handsome but are said to be sexually very frigid. When the women are eighteen or twenty, they choose boys in the pre-pubertal stage and bring them up to be their husbands.

MEAD:
You get that in parts of China where the child-nurse, the little girl who has been the nurse and therefore the surrogate mother of the baby boy, later becomes his wife.

HUXLEY:
I don't think this was an outgrowth of a nursemaid relation, I think it was the way they chose their men; in any case it must have a profound relation to this whole problem of differentiation of sexual identity.

LORENZ:
I have one question that came in my mind when you described the Tchambuli men with the ringlets, who giggled and so on. Quite a number of activities which we ascribe to femininity are in that case transferred en bloc to the other sex. On the other hand we find that certain single characteristics, which we in our culture call male or female, can be transferred separately to the other sex. Now I would be interested to go through all of your material to see which activities go to the other sex together and which activities occasionally singly; and here is the reason why I am interested in this: you know the old story which came up in our last meeting but one, about the relative sexuality in birds, where every sex can perform everything which is characteristic of the other sex, but en bloc. A raven or a jackdaw may behave as a male to a socially inferior partner or completely as a female to one ranking higher than itself in social order, and the sex of the partner does not matter in the least. But the two sets of male and female activities are never dissociated and never mixed. To one given partner the bird behaves either as a male or as a female. Interesting exceptions to this do take place when the social rank-relationship between two sexual partners becomes reversed, for instance if one of them is weakened by illness. J. Nicolai observed this in European bullfinches (*Pyrrhula europæa*): a male was slightly weakened by an illness and instantly the female switched to male activities and vice versa.

Now it seems to me I have to put my question by *reductio ad absurdum;* do you have any society where, let us say, the male is giggly and catty, as we put it, and at the same time strong and a fighter? The question is what is inseparably associated, and what can be transferred to the other sex.

MEAD:

We might find that there were key turning points—for example, the continuation of the falsetto voice might carry these other characteristics with it; or the handling of hair again might be sufficiently crucial so that it might carry other points with it. But I don't think I know of any society where you have women of the reproductive age with shaved heads in which you don't simultaneously have a diminution of femininity in general.

FREMONT-SMITH:

I wonder whether there is any indication in ethological studies that there is one leading character which the others follow.

LORENZ:

Well, with all these potentially ambivalent birds, dominance is the character which determines all others. The dominance relation of one bird to another will determine whether this bird feels 'male' towards his partner and 'female' to another.

FREMONT-SMITH:

And everything else goes with that?

LORENZ:

Everything goes with that; it is called a 'determopath'.

This refers again to a question that I had put to myself; you call certain characters masculine or male and then, when they appear in the other sex, too, you say that they are 'transferred' to that other sex. I wonder how much you are justified, from the ethological point of view, in calling these characters 'male', for short, and talking of 'transference of male characters'.

An interesting thing is that most of what we call 'male' in our culture would be male in the chimp and would be male in the greylag goose and would be male in the horse, and those female characters, cattiness, giggliness, coyness, are all typically female characters in chimps, horses and geese. What your American mother expects of male and female babies, respectively, are just the same, stereotype characters.

86

HUXLEY:

Yes, and if you look at this from a broad evolutionary point of view, you find that there *is* a greater frequency among males of dominance, large size, exploratory activity—all those things that we are accustomed to think of as masculine. But in a few cases, you get a total reversal, as with Phalaropes and Painted Snipe, and in a great number of cases you get sex equalization, either by both sexes looking and largely behaving like females, or by both sexes developing equivalent mutual display characters, and in that way behaving like males. This occurs in correlation with the mode of life of the species.

A rather important point is that these characters don't always go together in evolution. In species like the Grebes they go together—all the characters are equal in the two sexes, with minor quantitative differences; but in most song birds for instance, the male feeds the young but doesn't brood them: he's half feminine.

MEAD:

There are just one or two other aspects of this problem which I think might be relevant to our discussion. If we look at the way in which an infant is prepared to be an adult in any society, you will find societies in which both male and female infants are treated passively—so that the mother gives the food to the child, who is never expected to demand it; the child lies in a limp, relaxed way, is supported under her breast, is carried around in a net bag, and this passivity of course is a part of the relation between the mother and the child.

If the mother-child relationship has this great emphasis on passivity, then the first years of life, or the period when the child is carried and is breast fed, will have to be reversed later, and may have to be reversed very harshly.

On the other hand, both boys and girls may be treated as exceptionally active, as the Manus do for instance, where the child is encouraged to the highest degree of activity and the mother's breast is treated as a piece of plumbing entirely under the control of the child. Instead of the mother who takes her breast and gives it to the child in what is a complementary inter-personal relationship, you have a mother who happens to have a piece of rubber tubing attached to the front of her person, which happens to be connected with the milk, and the child grabs it, pulls it, pushes it, yanks it around, and you have a more or less continuous battle over it between the mother and the child; the mother isn't very comfortable and the breasts become elongated and unattractive very quickly, with the terrific batterings they take. Now when the children begin to eat, the parents start to stuff the child's mouth with food, and whereas in Bali this is the standard form of feeding which is passively accepted by the child, in Manus the child grabs the food away from the adult and gets a lump in each hand and feeds itself.

FREMONT-SMITH:
No sex differentiation at all?

MEAD:
No sex differentiation—this is true of both boys and girls.

Now traditional Manus culture involved putting very heavy social coercive taboos on girls later. This exceedingly active little girl was expected to go everywhere and do everything her brother did. She swam as well, she managed a canoe as well, she went where her father was, she expected to grab everything that she wanted and then when she was betrothed she had an enormous mat put over her head, and she was told that from then on she couldn't go anywhere where there were men, and had to stay with women—of whom she had a rather low opinion: they also had mats over their heads. It took very heavy sanctions to enforce this new behaviour.

There are all sorts of varieties of this kind of thing. Among the Bathonga in South Africa, for instance, at weaning the child is sent to the mother's village and indulged and played with, and allowed a great deal of licence—up to the time the little boy is about twelve, and then he is sent back home and the men put him through a perfectly terrible initiation ceremony to get him back into shape. One of the things we have to keep carefully focussed is events in the prefigurative phases of adult sexual life, all the way through from the way one sleeps, the way one is fed, and the way one is taught to walk, and the extent to which one is disciplined, and the degree to which these disciplines are appropriate for males or for females and the degree to which they are or are not differentiated between the two.

In the United States at present we have a period in which little girls are allowed to dress like little boys, which is the reversal of the European period where little boys were dressed so much more like girls. We have an early differentiation in clothes followed by—at about the eight-year- period—little girls all being allowed to put on blue jeans. It is a period when little girls flatly refuse to wear skirts, and there is just beginning now the ritual initiation ceremonies where children graduate from the eighth grade at about thirteen. In one of the famous experimental schools they started the evening in blue jeans, boys and girls dressed exactly alike, and then separated, and the girls went out and dressed in very pretty party dresses, the boys dressed in 'party' boys' clothes, and all came back and finished the evening with a dance. So that we see the development of a new ritual appropriate to handling this particular emphasis.

In any educational trend or in the examination of any social system in terms of sex roles, we have to remember that we don't know whether we get the greatest facilitation of growth by interference or non-interference. That is, you may agree with Gesell and Ilg's contention (Mead, 1947) that five is a much better age to start school than six, and conclude that in the United States we start children to school at the age when they are least prepared to go there. But we don't know whether starting children to school at the age they are best prepared to go there will produce the maximum effort or not. We don't know for instance whether the greatest degree of femininization of baby girls and masculinization of baby boys from birth would be the way to develop the bisexual capacities of each. There is considerable material that suggests that this doesn't develop whole human beings, that you don't develop the person as much if you over-develop the bipolarity between the two sexes.

There is one rather obvious comment that gets made on sex differences, and that is women deal with people, and men deal with things. Professor Zazzo said, for example, that little boys organize space better and have a greater interest in mechanical things, in things that are constructed. But it raises the question as to what, in different societies, is considered as things and what as people. In some societies, for instance, teaching is male; but when it is assigned to males then you may be dealing with public roles and there may be little discussion, little emphasis on certain types of human relations. Erik, do you want to make your point about the old Professor here? The point you were making last night about the fact that we permit the elderly professor to take a maternal role to some extent towards his student again?

ERIKSON:

Well, referring back to the puberty rites where the men behave in a certain ritualistic way as women, we said that this obviously had the meaning of telling the novitiates: from now on the group will be mother to you. We also said that this takes place in specific relation to the initiation into a new life stage, a clan, or certain occupations. I added privately my impression that in our specialized life, certain occupations take over that role. I thought of some such occupation as a professor who is permitted at least in some cultures a lesser degree of display of masculinity. He can wear longer hair and have a certain leaning toward, let us say, 'unmanly' interests.

FREMONT-SMITH:
It is respectable to be gentler. . . .

ERIKSON:
Gentler, more aesthetic, more impractical.

MEAD:
And this of course is true of the physician, as well as the professor, In other words, you have in the parent-child, in the mother-child, in the father-child, in the contrast between the sexes, a great set of models which may be used at any point in the institutional structure. The mother-child relationship may be repeated later between a man and an adolescent, or between a man and his wife. The whole institutional structure, when one looks at a society, can be analysed in terms of the recurrence of themes, with changes of sex roles very often, from one point to another. And we can't really understand the problem of personality or identity in any specific culture, without understanding the way in which at different periods in life, and in different occupational situations, one or another of these possible patterns of relationship can be used.

Sex Differences in Play Construction
of Twelve-year-old Children

ERIKSON:
Saturday morning lends itself well to an interlude between this week's and next week's discussions. I will present material from an investigation of sex differences in play construction of twelve-year-old children, which will continue our discussion of sex differences. At the same time, it will prepare the matter of clinical observation. These children were the subjects of a long-range developmental study. Almost twenty-five years ago, the parents of every third child born in Berkeley, California during a given period were asked to participate in a study made possible by a grant from the Rockefeller Foundation to the Institute of Child Welfare in the University of California. Dr. Jean Walker Macfarlane is the director of the study. I worked with her when the children were eleven, twelve and thirteen years old (they are now about twenty-five) and one of the procedures employed was that to be reported here.

Here, then, a new medium comes up for discussion. Such play observations as I will report today originate primarily in clinical work though I will reserve the discussion of clinical observation as such for next week. But I would like to tell you one brief clinical example in order to demonstrate the survival-value of play observation at any rate for the *therapist*. When I first came to America, I was asked to see a little boy of eight. His main symptom was soiling. This boy had been seen by a number of outstanding child psychiatrists, and they had not been able to find out what was wrong. There always came a moment in therapy when the boy would soil and stop responding to psychiatric questioning. Why? Not being able to understand his particular dialect too well, I started to play with him. Suddenly there was a gleam in his pale face, and he said, 'Let's play grocery store; I am the truck driver and you are the grocery man. I will deliver nuts to you.' 'Nuts' means crazy people—that much I had already learned in contact with American psychiatrists—so I became eager to see what he was going to 'deliver'.

He took plasticine, made balls of different sizes and different colours, and loaded a dump truck with them. Then he dumped the 'nuts' in the corner of the 'grocery store' which I had built for him. He took one big red ball and said 'This is Mummy nut'. Then he took a number of small red balls and said, 'These are the baby nuts' (I noticed that he took as many as there were children in his family). Then he took a big green ball and said, 'This is Uncle nut'. So I said to him 'Why does this family have an Uncle nut but not a Father nut?' At this point he soiled and left the room. The conclusion was obvious, that in his family there was an uncle, a somebody called an uncle, who was in the centre of what this boy had kept from his psychiatrists. This proved correct. His mother had told him, 'You can tell the psychiatrists everything, but if you tell them about the uncle, father will kill me'. But in play hieroglyphs, he could not help delivering the real 'nuts', in his family situation. This is not unconscious material, yet he did not realize that he had expressed it until my question made him aware of it. Such experiences, then, establish the clinical working hypothesis that, if you give an acutely troubled child play material to work with, the child will in play language in some way express his trouble, and this especially if you do not just listen to his words, but also watch the configurations of colour, size, arrangement, and so on. This is a statement on the *clinical* use of play, not on the nature of play. In other words, I want to disavow a 'traumatic' theory of play as such.

FREMONT-SMITH:

It seems to me highly important that when the child was asked the crucial question he didn't answer it, but instead had a vegetative response which he couldn't control, and defecated. This is an essentially psychosomatic situation in which the cortex cannot function and the lower centres are released, and you get a body-response which may be in behaviour or may be in a vegetative reaction.

ERIKSON:

Now in this case, and in others, play observation helps the therapy to survive even where full verbal communication fails. When I came to the Guidance Study in Berkeley the problem was different. I was not supposed to interview the children, because here the survival question was, how does one keep a long-range study together? There were parents who had trustingly given their children for two interviews every year, who had themselves come twice every year, who had let the children be photographed, tested, measured, and they had done this for the great Rockefeller Foundation and for the director of the study. The idea that their children would be exposed to a psychoanalyst, so it was felt, might be just one good thing too many. Here the study had to survive *me*. My work then consisted primarily in an attempt to take the data gathered on these twelve-year-old children, and to write a dynamic biography with a measure of prediction. My only systematic personal contact with the children consisted of a play method which was meant to give me one fresh impression in material to which my clinical eyes were accustomed. Each child, on three occasions half a year apart, would come into my room and find the following situation there.

There is a square table with a square blackboard of the same size. Any configuration built on this table will thus appear in an imaginary cube and have clear co-ordinates. Beside and behind this table there are two shelves with toys: blocks, people, cars and animals. There was no systematic selection of toys. I went to a toy store and bought what was available. In that sense (as in others) this cannot be called an experiment.

Now when the child came in I would say, 'I am interested in moving pictures. I would like to know what kind of moving pictures children would make if they had a chance to make pictures. Of course, I cannot provide you with a real studio and real actors and actresses; you will have to use these toys instead. Choose any of the things you see here and construct on this table an *exciting* scene out of an imaginary moving picture. Take as much time as you want and tell me afterwards what the scene is about.'

The children built their scenes and I sat at my desk. I sketched the intermediate stages, scenes that they built and then changed or replaced, and noted how they seemed to go about their task, and their whole attitude towards the play. At the end I asked one question: 'What is the most exciting thing in this scene?' This was necessary because often when I looked at the final scene, there was nothing obviously exciting. In the case of a girl, there may be a living room, a little girl playing the piano and the family listening to her; or in boys, there is traffic on the street, there is a policeman, everything is quiet. There seems often to be almost an amnesia for my suggestion that something exciting should be presented. At the end of the procedure I would tell them that the scene was very nice, and they would leave. Then I would photograph the scene.

While this was not the purpose of the study, gradually I received a definite impression of sex differences. I blotted out the 'M's' and

'F's' on the little identification tags which can be seen in the pictures, and give the scenes of seventy-five boys and seventy-five girls to two advanced graduate students, one man and one woman, with a list of block configurations. The problem was: could they identify my criteria for particular block configurations, such as a simple enclosure, a building, a bridge, a street crossing, and so on, and then could they rate each picture for the presence and absence of such configuration. This statistical procedural basis was published in two papers. (Erikson 1951, Honzik 1951.)

Now as I show you some pictures, I wish you would pay attention to whether there are blocks at all, or whether there aren't; if there are blocks, whether they make for high buildings or low buildings, whether the buildings are open or closed, whether the whole construction is in the foreground or in the background; and whether the buildings contain people and animals or are surrounded by people and animals. The sex differences lie in these simplest spatial relationships.

FIG. 1

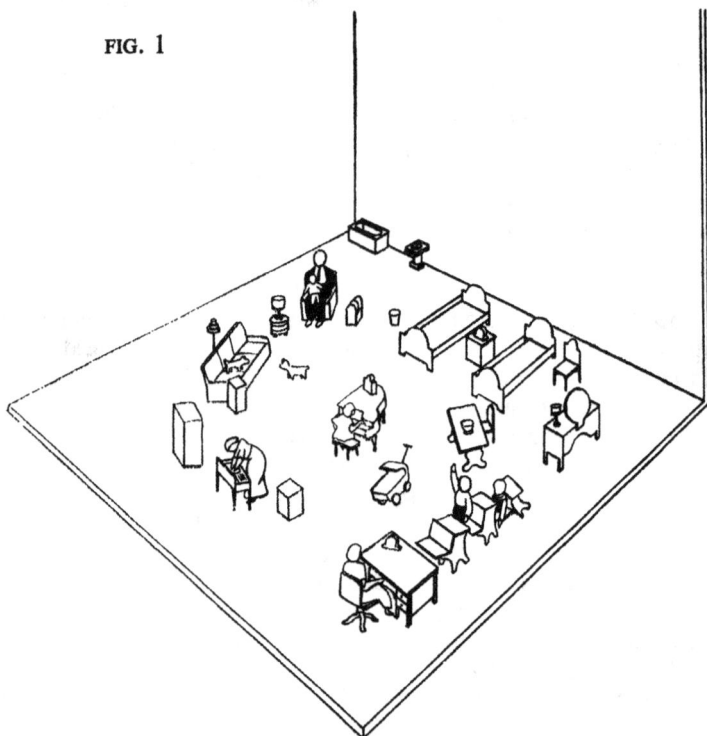

Fig. 1, I would classify as an open interior. There are no walls around the house, nor walls separating the different rooms of the house. This is a kind of construction which occurs significantly more often in girls' scenes.

HUXLEY:
This kind of construction represents a number of rooms for different functions, study and sleep and so forth though, doesn't it?

ERIKSON:
Yes, but without walls. There is a study, a kitchen, a bedroom. Within the 'typical' configuration there was usually a 'unique' element, which would lead me further into the history of the child. Such unique elements I will point out later.

FREMONT-SMITH:
Did you know the history of the child before she came in?

ERIKSON:
I knew some of it, but I would take a fresh look after the play construction because of that clinical working hypothesis—that if you give a child space to play with, she will not only be playful in a variety of ways, i.e. express mastery, but also indicate what she has not mastered entirely. I may add in this case that the distribution of the toys over the whole table I have come to consider a sign of good balance in a child. Later on I will show you some examples of constructions which are entirely built against the wall, or entirely out in one corner, in which case a particular strain can be assumed.

INHELDER:
Was the child talking while playing?

ERIKSON:
No. Most children would not, until they said, 'I am finished'.

FREMONT-SMITH:
The majority of these children became sufficiently preoccupied so that they worked silently?

ERIKSON:
Yes. In fact, the degree of concentration was really surprising. 'Conflict' may be too strong a word, but to see a twelve-year-old put a chair there, or a block, and then pause, and then take it away

and put something else there—you could feel that the spatial task had a peculiar fascination.

INHELDER:
Very young children are absolutely unable to work and play without talking; verbal and manual activities in the beginning are intimately related.

ERIKSON:
Yes. This is one reason among many why a transition would have to be made in any developmental study between the age when the child would prefer to play on the floor, or would play with the toys without the aim of a final construction, and the age when the children would be able to 'construct' silently. This was *constructing* and not play in the sense of toying, handling, or manipulating with running commentary.

FREMONT-SMITH:
Would you say that these twelve-year-olds a good part of the time were sufficiently preoccupied that they lost their awareness of you as an observer?

ERIKSON:
In an overt sense, yes: in the vast majority of cases they paid no attention to me. However, I have the impression that a thorough analysis would find references to the observer both in the content and in the spatial arrangement.

BOWLBY:
Of course there is always a communication because you have asked them to communicate.

ERIKSON:
Yes; a communication condensed into a completed construction with a theme. If one compared the verbal output that appeared at the end of these play constructions with that in Rorschach tests, or TAT tests, it was remarkable how, in this case, the energy of confabulating was apparently absorbed by the activity of constructing and how very brief were the stories told at the end. In fact, I often had the feeling that the children often told me 'just anything' and that the important thing was in the arranging.

96

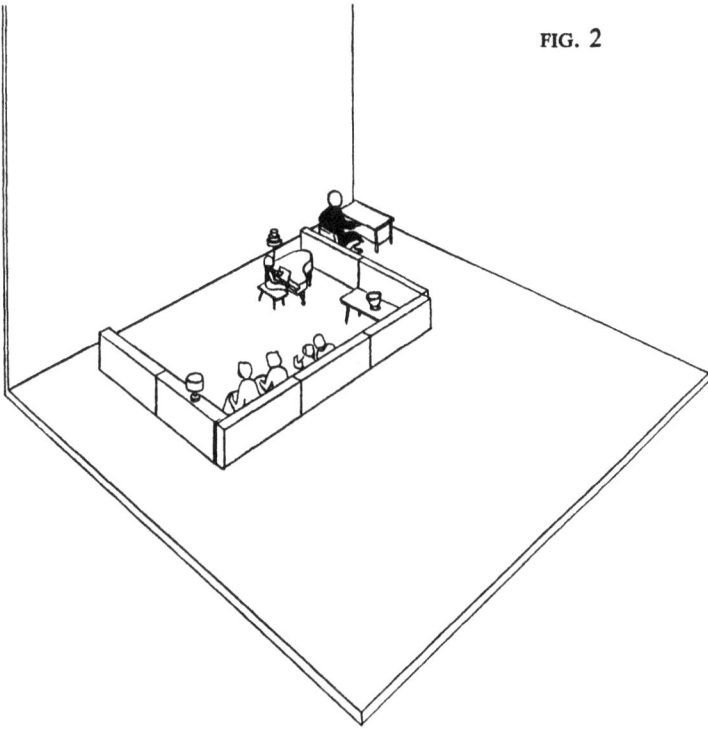

FIG. 2

Fig. 2 is what I would call a 'low enclosure'. A low enclosure is one that is only one block high, has no ornaments, no roof, no tower, but on occasion an 'elaborate front door'. This again is on the whole a feminine construction. Boys build such enclosures primarily in connexion with more complicated structures. In this case, the low enclosure is attached to the background, in fact, it opens up toward the wall.

TANNER:

These are all twelve-year-olds, aren't they? Some had reached menarche and some had not, I take it. Was there any difference between pre- and postmenarcheal?

ERIKSON:

I undertook one preliminary study with our paediatrician on the appearance of a particular play configuration which seemed to have

G   97

a relationship to the appearance of the sesamoid bone in the hand (which in turn is related to the menarche). There was a definite relationship.

GREY WALTER:
What is the number of children?

ERIKSON:
In this play study there were 150—75 boys and 75 girls.

TANNER:
All twelve years old?

ERIKSON:
Eleven, twelve or thirteen—the children came twice a year so it was either the end of the eleventh year, the twelfth year or the beginning of the thirteenth. Today I am not differentiating between chronological ages but refer to the overall maturational stage of pre-puberty.

INHELDER:
Then you have two or three samples from each child?

ERIKSON:
Yes.

BOWLBY:
Was there any essential difference between the first, the second and the third presentation?

ERIKSON:
Overt differences, very much so. But often with a theme that goes through all of one child's constructions.

LORENZ:
I was going to ask the opposite question. Was there a significant similarity or identity for the same child in the three constructions?

ERIKSON:
Overt similarity, in some. Identity of themes in most. I will illustrate this later.

Sufficiently so that you could say of any one of them: I recognize this as. . . .

No. Only when I analysed them would I see what theme ran through. Maybe after having analysed a few hundred more I would learn to recognize individual styles.

FIG. 3

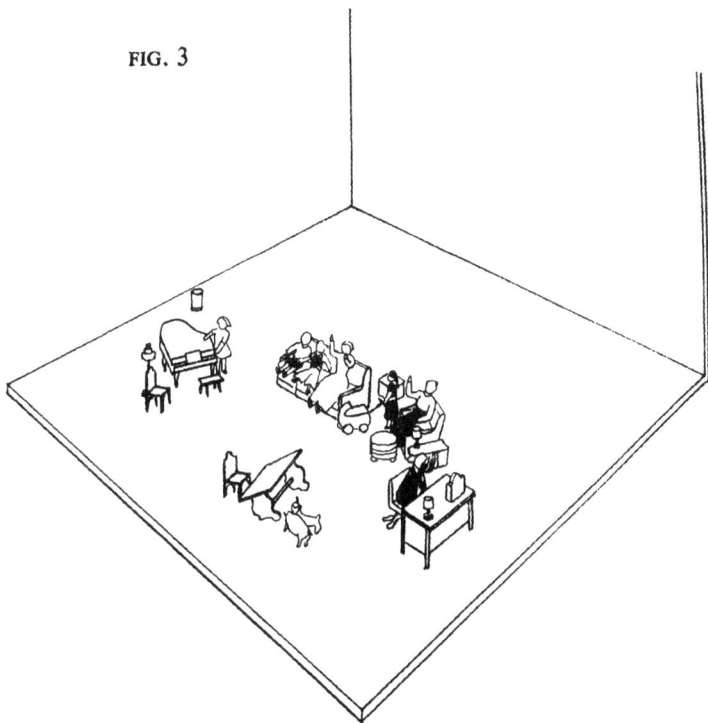

Fig. 3 is a very feminine configuration. Not only are there no walls, but a round arrangement of furniture, with either an animal or a male breaking into the circle. Sometimes both appear—such as father coming home on a lion and right behind him, upholding a semblance of law and order, a policeman. The Fig. 3 configuration was done by an Italian-American girl. You see how visibly excited that family is. The child spent quite some time turning their arms up in the air. The exciting thing is that a little pig has run into the

99

family house, and in this case it is not the policeman, but the dogs who are trying to protect the house.

HUXLEY:

Coming in also?

ERIKSON:

So it seems. I might mention that after a while I became so used to sex differences that it disturbed me when a boy did something which I thought only girls did. There was one boy who built such a scene of a round configuration of furniture, he had a whole row of wild animals march into the house. This boy said 'Goodbye', went to the door, stopped, and said, 'There is something wrong', turned around, and rearranged the animals on a tangent to the circle, walking by, not into the house. Do you think he had noticed that I thought there was something wrong, telepathy, I mean? At any rate he was one of the only two boys who ever produced such a configuration.

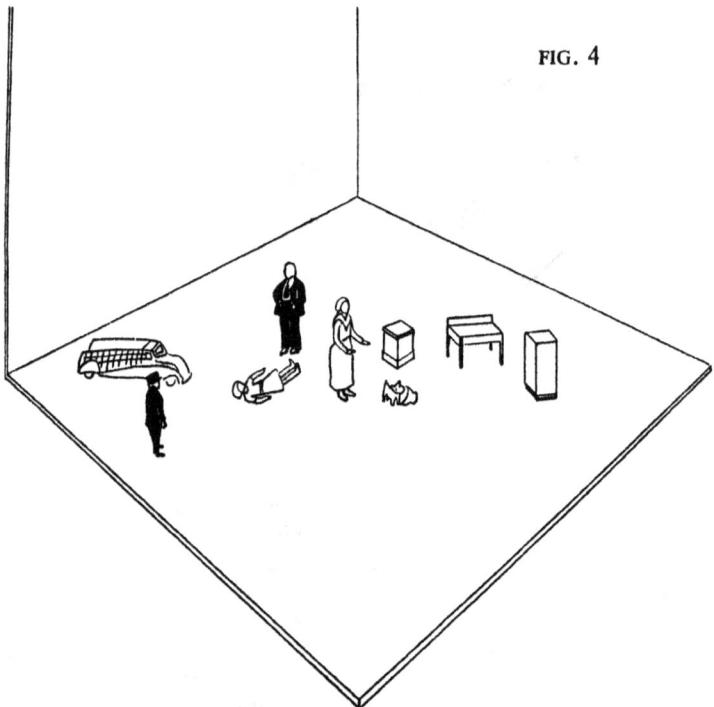

FIG. 4

Fig. 4 is also a feminine configuration: there is a lack of differentiation between indoors and outdoors. A home scene (a little dog overturns a bowl) and a traffic accident fused into one another without any differentiation of indoors and outdoors.

ZAZZO:
Is the surface on which you build always the same size?

ERIKSON:
Yes, certainly.

HUXLEY:
The diagonal arrangement in Fig. 4 is curious—does it represent anything? Some tension between something or other?

ERIKSON:
Yes, indeed, a conflict between staying close to the wall and wishing to get away from it. It has to do with tension over emancipation from the mother. It is as if the accident would indicate 'You had better stay close'—while the little dog represents mischievousness.

LORENZ:
I was a very strictly brought up child, and I distinctly remember a time when I was just allowed to take walks by myself, to go hunting, and to go fishing alone. And then I never went on trodden pathways, but always in diagonals across the fields. I can definitely remember that this was to prove my own independence.

ERIKSON:
Fig. 5 is a girl's high enclosure, with only one ornamental block— and that is on the gate. Again, the opening is toward the back wall. Inside there is a bullfight which the family watches.
Now we come to the boys. The policeman is of all people the figure used most in the boys' constructions, twice as often as the cowboy, for example, who certainly in Western America is an outstanding image of identification. But there is an exclusively masculine scene at this age—just traffic and a policeman to guard it. This does not need illustration.

101

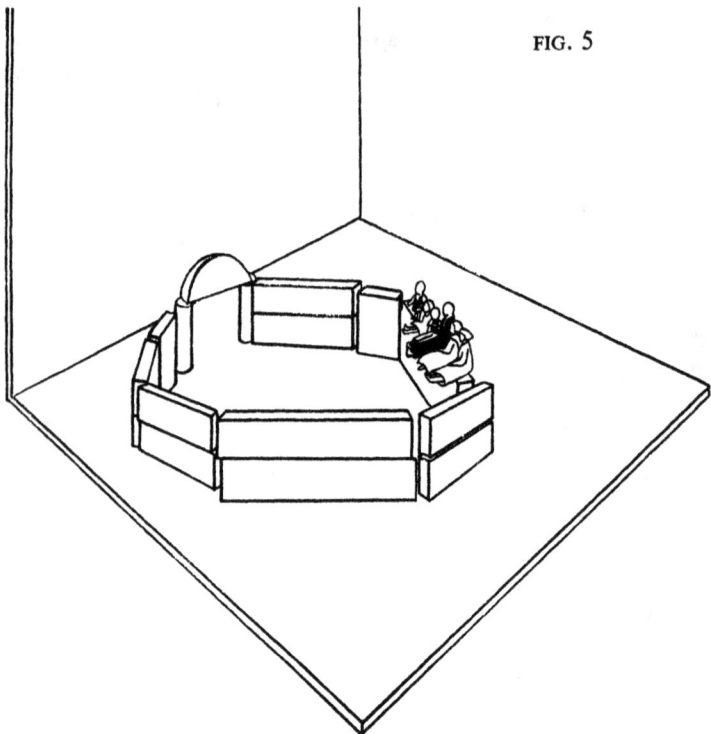

FIG. 5

GREY WALTER:
You had cowboys available?

ERIKSON:
Yes, and Indians.

Fig. 6 is a boy's construction: a locomotive constructed out of blocks. I would definitely call this an 'elaborate building', and as a building it is a very masculine construction. Yet, when I asked the boy 'What is so exciting about it?' he said that is a very, very narrow bridge, which that train has to squeeze through. This boy had an acute and painful phimosis. Thus what dominates at the moment as a discomfort or a conflict enters by way of a unique detail in what otherwise is a normal and in fact outstanding performance.

Fig. 7 is a typical boy's construction. There is an Indian who wants to attack a fort, which, as you see, has many guns. Boys, more often than girls, erect buildings, cover them with roofs, provide them with ornaments and other items which stick out: towers, guns, etc.

102

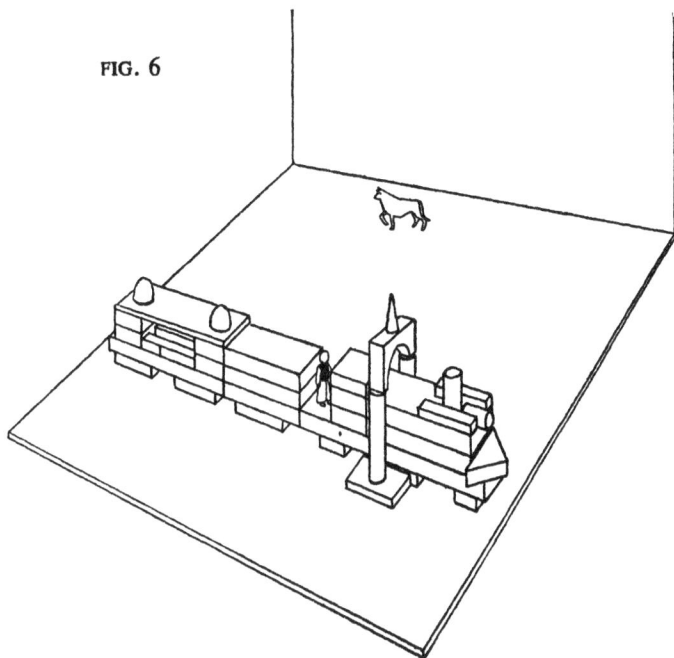

FIG. 6

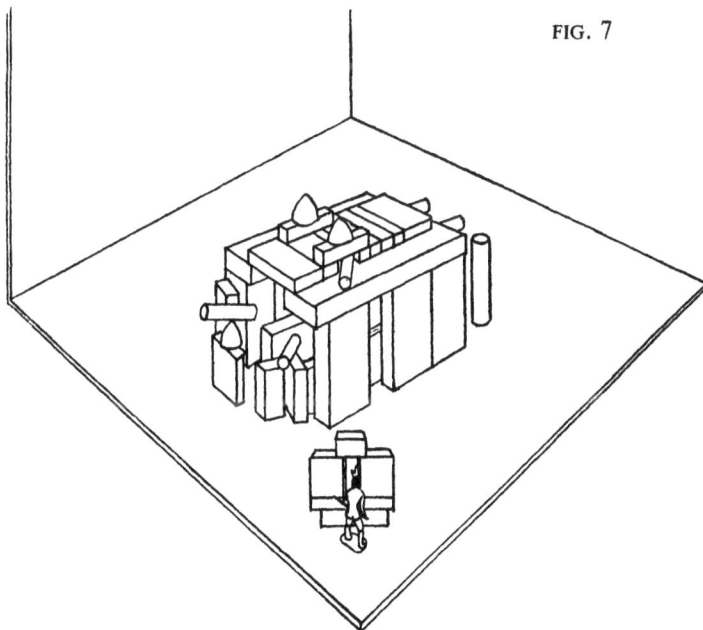

FIG. 7

DE SAUSSURE:

Why is it typically masculine, because after all it's something rather closed in and there isn't any traffic?

ERIKSON:

It is typically masculine because it is the erection of a complicated structure. This configuration can occur together with traffic or it can alternate with traffic. I will later on list together the various criteria for masculine and feminine.

FIG. 8

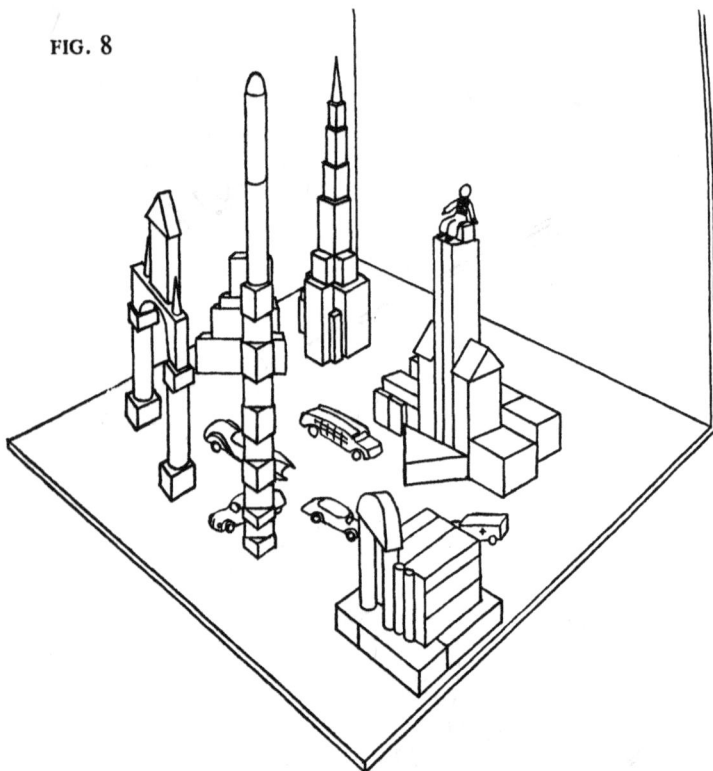

I do not need to point out that Fig. 8 is a boy's construction. It is almost too masculine. It isn't just height that is masculine. In connexion with the highest towers and buildings there is in the exciting or unique element a downward trend, as if such height went too far. He 'stuck his neck out'. In this case, the exciting element is that the proud boy sitting on top of the world is really insane, and in fact, on top of a sanatorium.

FREMONT-SMITH:
 He said that?

ERIKSON:
 Yes. Some of the highest buildings are counteracted by some downfall, some danger. I asked another boy who built the very highest tower, 'What is the exciting thing about this?' he said, 'You must not touch it. It is built in such a way that it would collapse, if you touch it.' I might add that ruins, that is buildings that have broken down, are exclusively male, with one exception which I will show you later.

HUXLEY:
 In Fig. 8 the gateway is very like the feminine gateway you showed before. Do boys frequently add that to their constructions?

ERIKSON:
 Yes, there are, of course, low enclosures, gateways, and other 'female' configurations in boys, but they are mostly in conjunction with a high building. In this construction, the gate is actually that of a bank and the 'insane' boy had tried to break into it. Thus the gate is part of an intrusive theme, which leads to the downfall.

RÉMOND:
 Do you allow the child a fixed time to build what he wants to show you, or do you give him as long as he likes?

ERIKSON:
 It is not fixed.

HUXLEY:
 How long was it usually?

ERIKSON:
 Anywhere from two minutes to half an hour. Some children would get it over with very quickly, and get out, though not without leaving some message which would indicate their motivation for this. The only child who entirely refused to build a construction, and said that it was all too childish a task was the smallest child in the study. I think she, too, got her message across.
 We now have enough elements available to decipher just a few more complicated statements.

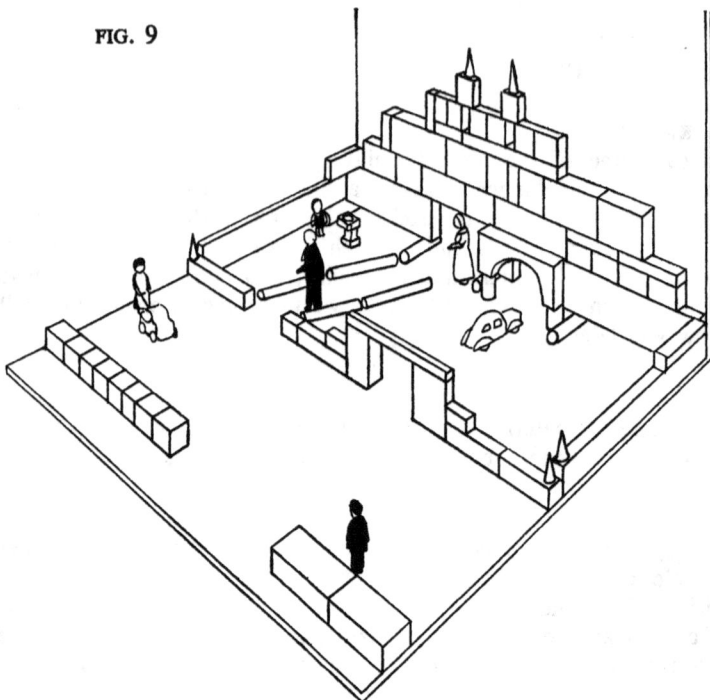
FIG. 9

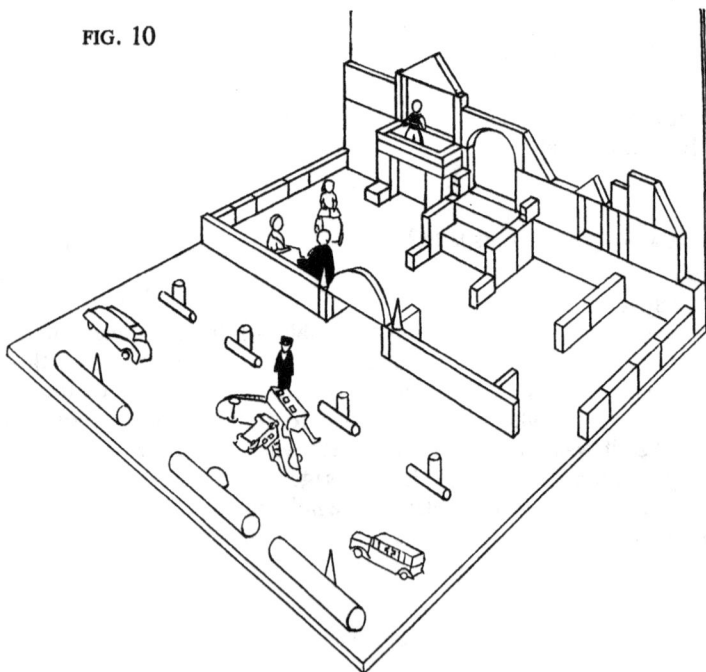
FIG. 10

Fig. 9 is by a boy who at the time was highly dependent on his mother, and with a certain 'façade' of aloofness. This is expressed by a high façade, leaning against the background. But not only that. When I asked him 'What is the exciting element?' he said that this man (the 'father') has placed some bombs underneath that façade. You can see the cylinders. So here again, his high façade, if you pushed slightly, would collapse. But now let's see how such a theme may develop as time passes.

Fig. 10 shows his later construction, again a façade, this time well founded, but still against the background. The boy standing there, high and mighty. The same cylinders which before had represented bombs are now out here, each one kept by a peg from rolling towards the building. So he has regained safety. I cannot go now into that critical year in the family history.

FREMONT-SMITH:
He has regained safety, but he has not forgotten the danger?

ERIKSON:
He has 'displaced' it. Yes.

LORENZ:
My only objection is that it is too beautiful!

ERIKSON:
I know—it was my objection too for a long time.
Fig. 11 you may also find too good to be true. Here is the only child whose mother came in with her. I had to ask the mother to wait outside.
This child builds a boardwalk against the back wall, and another one coming out into space. Not a diagonal then, but two separate tendencies, to hang on to the background and to come out. Let me show how the repetition of a theme underlines this configuration. Here is a cowboy guarding a bull. Here is a policeman guarding a bear, a tiger and a lion. Here is an Indian guarding the baby. So that you see that in content and form the emphasis is on the 'Mother watches over me, I hang on to her'. In this particular case, attempt at a symbiosis with the mother was clinically evident.
Incidentally, only two children ignored the table altogether. One was this girl, the other a very meek little coloured boy. He built under the table. He nearly made me cry. He didn't dare to build where the others did.

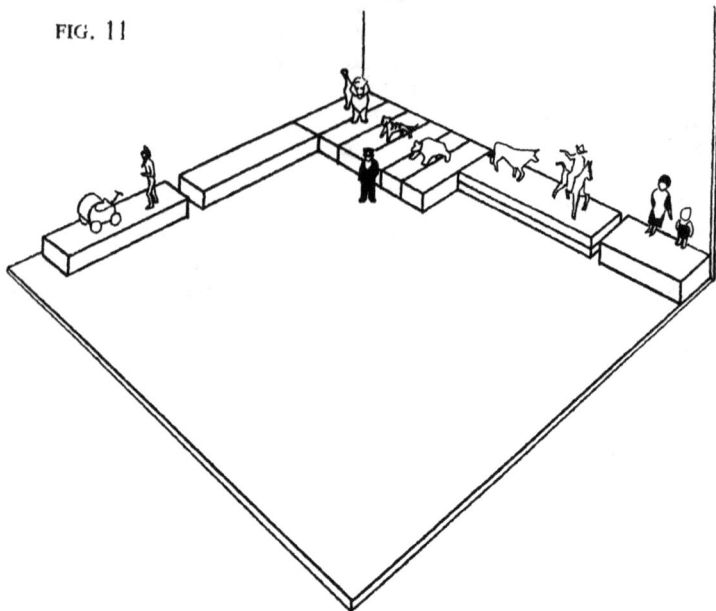

FIG. 11

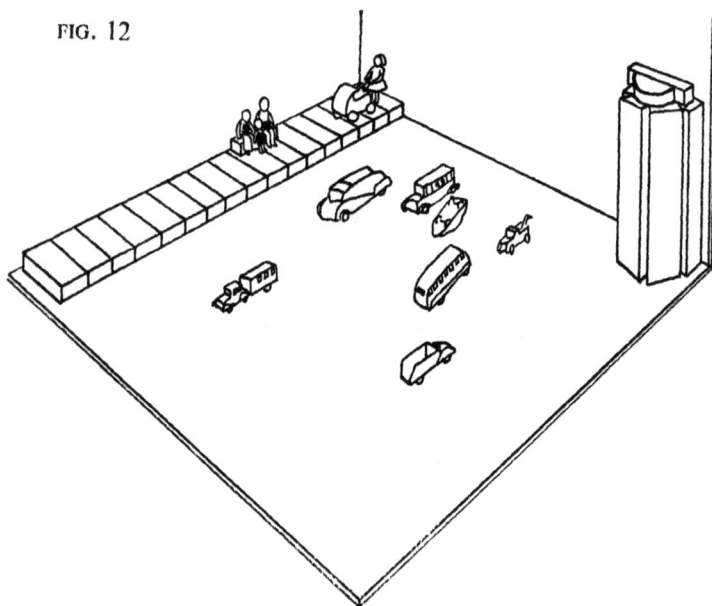

FIG. 12

Fig. 12 is the construction made by the same girl half a year later. The conflict over emancipation from the mother is now more clearly counterpointed. There is a 'tower', hugging the background, and there is a board-walk reaching out, and the children sit and watch the world go by. Such changes in configuration often correspond to clear-cut changes in the interview material secured by other workers. Incidentally, the only high towers built by girls are in the back third of the table, and the highest tower built by any girl was built on the shelf back behind the table.

Fig. 13 is an example of the development of one theme during one session. This boy was an enuretic. He started with this phallic tower out in the foreground. Then he took the tower down. His configuration then went downwards and backwards to Fig. 14. He moved it into the background, and made it a low enclosure such as is typical for girls. At the same time, his final story 'regressed', as it were, for it concerned a sleeping baby.

HUXLEY:
Was this in the same interview?

ERIKSON:
Yes. In later constructions he overcame these trends. Here in Fig. 15 is his brother, at the time more 'outgoing' and more masculine. The similarity of initial configuration is uncanny. I do not believe that he could have possibly known what his brother had built. He starts with a phallic tower of more moderate height. But then (Fig. 16) he builds outward, retaining the tower, and adds what I call a 'barrier'—an exclusively male configuration. By the same token his story is concrete and up-to-date: this represents the entrance to the San Francisco World's Fair.

Let me now try and summarize the masculine variables and the feminine ones. The channelization of traffic through tunnels and street crossings is masculine and so is the erection of elaborate and high structures. To this corresponds the theme of the policeman who arrests dangerous motion, and the theme of a downward trend which counteracts excessive height. Then, on the other hand, simple walls which merely enclose interiors are feminine, with an emphasis by ornamentation on the vestibular access to the interior. Interiors without walls are feminine. So is the intrusion into such an interior of a dangerous or mischievous animal or male creature. On the other hand, the peaceful scene, say of a girl playing the piano for the family, is also a typically female 'exciting scene'. Enclosing a space

109

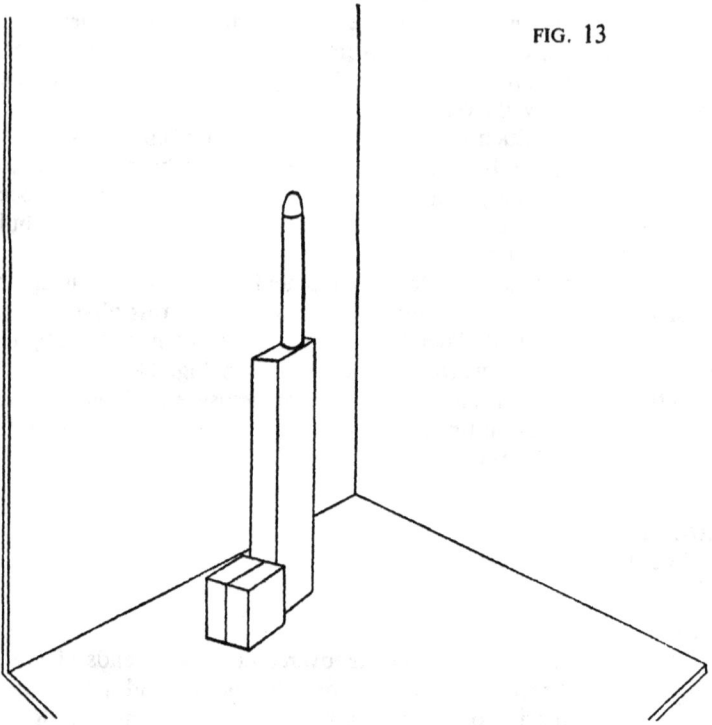

FIG. 13

FIG. 14

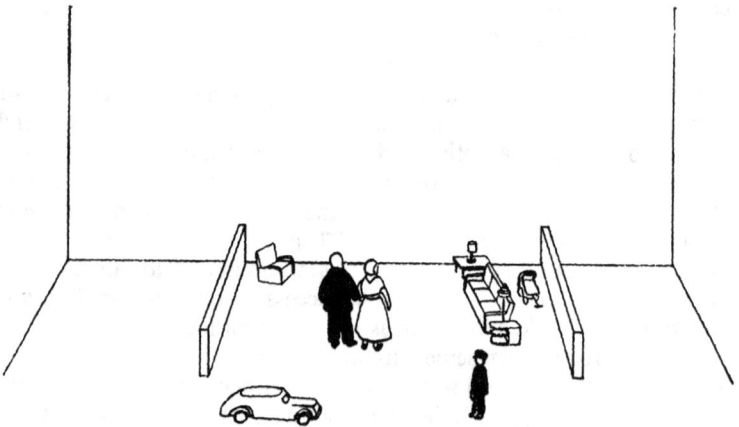

110

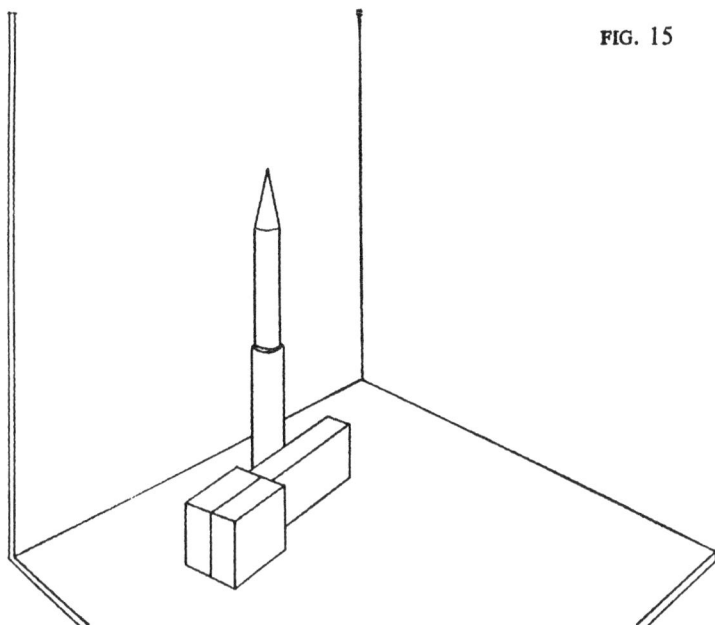

FIG. 15

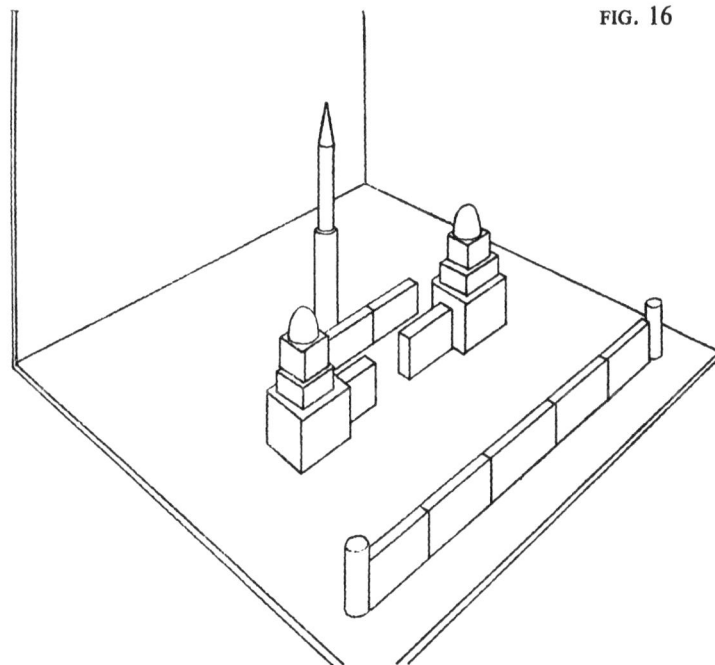

FIG. 16

with three or four low walls is such a common procedure that you have to specify whether or not such an enclosure appears in conjunction with high buildings, whether it is enclosing things, or is surrounded by things.

Without prejudging the discussion, one basic fact can be stated now, namely the analogy between the sex differences in play-configurations and the primary physiological sex-differences, that is in the male the emphasis on the external, the erectable, the intrusive, and the mobile—in the female, on the internal, on the vestibular, on the static, on what is contained and endangered in an interior. You will recognize immediately that these are all configurations which in Margaret Mead's material appeared in manifold cultural elaborations. Contrary to what some of you may think in an analyst looking at his material, these differences came as a surprise to me, having leaned toward a kind of anthropological relationism at the time. The age at which the play constructions were done perhaps determines the closeness of these themes to physiological facts. At ages eleven, twelve, thirteen changes in the sex organs as well as overall sex impulses must enter at least the preconscious awareness of the child. Whether this has to do more with actual information, by direct observation, or with a particular kinaesthetic tension, or with instinctual drives or something else—this I will leave for the discussion.

zazzo:
What always bothers me with psychoanalytic explanations like those you gave us just now is that the symbolism is too direct and too close. For example, the wall which would symbolize the need to lean on the mother—couldn't it really express a much more general fact, of which the seeking for the mother's support is an extremely important aspect for the child, but only one aspect: the lack of confidence, the desire for support is something much more general, even, than the need for the mother. The phenomenon of 'sticking to' or 'closing' has been observed in small children. In the drawings of children up to three years we see that the copy is made directly on top of the model, they adhere to the model, they construct on top of the model and they are not yet capable of measuring space or disassociating themselves from space. Among the patients observed by Mayer Gross and among the hypoxic people that we observed ourselves there was a regression to this attitude of sticking to the model. You notice it for example in the Porteus mazes: our patients stick to the model and they can't get out of the mazes again. I think we are dealing with a very general phenomenon showing at

various levels the subject's difficulty of autonomous expression. In the small child this phenomenon is so obviously linked to the need for the mother that I think it would be dangerous to consider automatically that the keeping close to walls is a hanging on to the mother. I see the mother as a particular case, extremely important, but which cannot furnish the principle explaining this general attitude.

ERIKSON:
I think that your observations support my point. I used the word 'mother' to connote one image of dependency among many, and yet the original model of what one was 'attached' to. The fact that sick people would show a tendency to 'adhere', and, as you said, to 'regress' would give one the right to say that these people wish to lean on somebody in a way which is modelled on the original need for maternal protection. In my material, I would add that I had at my disposal ten years of observations made by others and ratings by other workers. It is true, of course, that these ratings did not always concern a lasting manifest and conscious mother-dependence. Often such a dependence is sporadic, latent, and unconscious, and must be inferred from behaviour and from projective tests. So, if I say that there was a coincidence between spatial tendency in play and some kind of mother-dependence in life, this is not a symbolic judgement. All the same, I would conclude that to accept a wall as a symbol of a mother in imaginative material opens up much to our understanding which would otherwise remain hidden.

My reference to 'mother' was not intended as a full causal explanation. I think this has been imputed to me rather on the basis of what an analyst is expected to do. I described something and I pointed to a configurational relationship.

ZAZZO:
You spoke of mothers and it seems to me you spoke explicitly of mothers when one gets close to a wall. Now since yesterday I have had a bad foot because I twisted it and I go along holding on to the wall. Is it the need for my mother that makes me hang on to the wall because I twisted my foot and why did I twist my foot?

ERIKSON:
Well, of course, in reality walls are not mothers, mothers not walls, and a *mal au pied* is only deplorable. But in imaginative material, a wall can symbolize maternal protection. I would claim a right to use such a symbol in an individual dream or play-act, if

the associative material supports it. Here, the probability is supported by a comparison of these children by independent observers.

PIAGET:

As regards space I should like to say a word on the difference between boys and girls. We find differences as regards space in all kinds of connexions and not only in games. For example, in the results of factorial analysis, the spatial factor is better represented among boys than among girls. On the other hand, in experiments on perception we generally get better results—that is less pronounced systematic errors—among boys than among girls. As regards space representation I think that Mlle Inhelder would agree with me —it is true that we have not carried out systematic studies on the differences in the sexes—that there too the boys are slightly advanced in relation to girls. I note then a difference as regards cognitive functions (perception and intelligence). You show this, moreover, from the affective point of view in the symbolism of play. There are complex relations between the two kinds of fields. It is very possible that we are dealing with transformations that are simultaneously affective and intellectual. I myself would certainly think so. But it is also possible that one of the factors involves the other and I know psychoanalysts who consider that it is the affective factor which constitutes the primordial one and that this leads to intellectual transformations. I think personally that there are here a series of correlated factors without one factor dominating the other, because the affective (or energetic) aspect and the cognitive (or structural) aspect of behaviour are always interdependent and inseparable.

HUXLEY:

I was going to make a rather similar observation. That boys are more interested in mobility, in traffic and in the outer world, and that, as we heard yesterday, they are more mechanically inclined, are obviously correlated, as you say, with their own anatomy, but is it necessary to think that there is only one cause of this? Is there not also perhaps a higher tonicity and a greater interest in manipulation, and these then get focused on their anatomy, and the two reinforce each other and build up a complex structure?

ERIKSON:

I think that these sex differences are less symbolic than they are the experimental stuff out of which symbolism emerges. Now, in spite of my instruction to present an 'exciting scene from an imaginary

114

moving picture', little of the kind was produced. These children go to moving pictures once or twice a week. In 450 constructions there were very few motion-picture scenes, and there were hardly any dolls who were named after famous motion-picture stars of the kind that are on the billboards, in the press, and actually on the walls of the children's rooms.

Next, take the actual aspirations of the children. The cowboy was used much less than the policeman. There was an aviator figure available, and at that time, there was an enormous stepping-up of armament in the air. Some elder brothers of our boys and many of the boys themselves, at that time, wanted to become aviators. But the aviator figure was chosen only a little more than the figure of the monk. There were toy automobiles. For the young girls as well as the young boys in California, the wish to drive and some day own an automobile is very important. In fact, Margaret said something yesterday about the automobile already becoming more or less an accessory of the American female, while the airplane becomes the symbol of the executive male. This has an interesting sociological counterpart in the fact that in California it is now the girls who ride horses, and that many boys consider it effeminate to be a passionate horse-lover. Nevertheless, the girls in these constructions use much fewer automobiles and horses. All of this would make it difficult to come to any simple sociological explanation for the preferences shown here. The use of space and of things moving in it seems to serve more basic 'play-tendencies'.

INHELDER:
Have you also found appreciable differences in terms of age in the way children represent these scenes? Do the youngest ones take more elements from immediate reality, whereas the older ones elaborate the events symbolically? We have observed during imaginary games between several children facts which, at first sight, seemed contradictory. Emotionally well-balanced children of five to eight years, playing in groups of three, improvised imaginary games whose elements reproduced fairly faithfully their daily life, whereas those of eight to ten years seemed to take a very special pleasure in making up symbolic scenes (every symbolic game of course pre-supposes a certain amount of fiction). This late symbolic development is no doubt due to the difficulty experienced by children in· improvising symbolic scenes involving several children. Have you noted similar differences in your individual symbolic games or have you, on the contrary, noted a development in the opposite direction, going from pure fiction to a more faithful copy of reality?

115

ERIKSON:

I know the play of smaller children only in clinical situations. It was obvious that in these constructions girls, more often than boys, would immediately put people together, a trend which may correspond to what Margaret said yesterday about the woman's closer relationship to people in preference to things and ideas.

GREY WALTER:

Could I ask a rather general question? I wonder whether you could help those of us who lack background training in the field of psychoanalysis to assimilate these very rich titbits of information, by suggesting how we could regard them from the standpoint of the theory of communication? The first thing I personally should like to have defined would be the noise-level and the band-width of the channel through which you and the children are communicating. This play of theirs is essentially a language. But in my case the channel is of unknown band-width—I don't know how many bits of information can be conveyed per second, I don't know how rich a language it is. I haven't yet gathered how many things the child could do. And I don't know the noise-level—I don't know how much randomness there is in the choice of the items the child used.

ERIKSON:

I have described how the child comes in, and how the child finds on these few shelves a great number of blocks of all sizes and shapes. . . .

GREY WALTER:

Always in the same position, equally accessible for each child?

ERIKSON:

Oh, yes. Rearranged after each child leaves, in the same way, except that of course the blocks are lying in a heap, the small blocks by themselves, and the big blocks by themselves, and the ornamental items by themselves. Then the toys are arranged in boxes, but, as I said, they were toys of all sizes, materials and colour. Since I had no principle on which I could standardize I just took what I found.

FREMONT-SMITH:

About how many toys were there?

ERIKSON:

I would say about ten cars; and there was an airplane, which was almost never used. There was a little family, father, mother, a boy of let us say fifteen, a girl of twelve, a little girl of six, and a little boy of five, and a baby. These were German dolls, and came in a box, and were beautifully done and could be bent. Some of the other toys could not be bent. The policeman was a lead figure and so was the aviator.

Speaking of communication, I would like briefly to add something which may not refer to Grey Walter's question. But I cannot deny a feeling that not everybody would get such constructions from children. If one is used to eliciting information from people I think one behaves differently than if one wonders if they are going to give or not. In the way I invited the child to perform, I may have expressed that I expected something pretty good here. Afterwards, I was myself very much impressed with the fact that much of this was too good to be true. Maybe my clinical experience made me select the right combination of stimuli. The procedure has been repeated once by some other workers on a large scale with college students, and the results were disappointing. But when I asked, 'Did you give instructions?' the psychologists said, 'Our instructions were like yours. We asked them "Build on this paper the most *traumatic* scene of your childhood"!' That explained, of course, the fact that the students immediately shrank and did the most conventional things, carefully hiding anything that might have been traumatic. In my work with college students I used the instruction to produce a *dramatic* scene out of an imaginary play.

FREMONT-SMITH:
Nobody else tried your instructions with these children? So that you are the only sort of receptor for the material? It has been brought out again and again in such simple things as taking an IQ on a child, that the relationship established may make an enormous difference in the IQ result. One would expect that the children would feel at once that someone has a natural understanding of them and that they would be freer and bring out material which they might not bring out to someone who did not have an equally receptive understanding.

MEAD:
I think it is also important in connexion with Grey's question to point out that these objects are all highly culturally patterned. Blocks of this sort have been made for children in western European and American culture for a long time, and they represent a crystalliza-tion of age-long symbolism. The fact that you can't bend a police-man might also be regarded as symbolic. All the objects are very

highly standardized. We can compare this with Margaret Lowen-feld's world game, where she has made a systematic attempt to get all possible relevant material. That is, if the towns have lamp-posts in them, then there is a lamp-post in the test, and so forth. She is attempting to present the child with a vocabulary range that is very wide, whereas what Erik was doing was giving them just enough material with which to react. Now when I use play materials I restrict them a great deal more still. A doll, a snake and a teddy bear, for instance, is a very good combination. You can do almost everything with it, and you don't want much more, if what you want is to get a general pattern rather than individual differences.

GREY WALTER:

I like to think of these observations as linguistic ones, because they are using at least a culturally determined vehicle in the same class as a language, which one can define in terms of letters, syllables, phonemes and so forth. Do you consider the elements with which you provide the children (approximately twenty elements apart from the blocks which are the punctuation marks and spaces in the language, so to speak) as letters or as words? For example, can these elements make nonsense? If a child says a word, that obviously has a meaning, it has a semantic content, but a letter has no semantic content, except some single letters like 'a' and 'I' in English and so on.*

*Reading through this discussion I feel that these clinical methods could be enormously improved if they were planned and analysed as problems in Communication Theory. Unfortunately, this is beyond my competence but I would refer to the first Gospel in the New Testament of Communication, the *Mathematical Theory of Communication* by Claude Shannon & Warren Weaver (1949). As an example of this approach to linguistic problems, one can synthesize sentences mechanically in English by working out the transition probabilities of words and phrases as they are actually used. This means that given, say, the word 'there' to start with, the most likely next word statistically is 'is'. Proceeding cumulatively in this way the following sentence was in fact generated purely mechanically —I believe it was the first coherent spontaneous utterance by a machine: 'There is no reverse gear on a motor cycle'. This statement is not only syntactically admissible, it also happens to be true, and, what is more, could be considered analytically of great significance as coming from a machine, for it implies perhaps —'in a system which maintains equilibrium by continuous motion, stability is obtained by sacrificing reversibility; creatures that require inherent stability must accept the condition that time has an arrow pointing to the grave'. This nonsense is in the Lewis Carroll category because it should make one think more carefully, in this case about the probable significance of statements and behaviour such as Erik was describing; to what extent is their content dependent on transitional or structural probabilities; which of these probabilities are culturally and which individually determined? Can one devise a system in which these questions would be answered explicitly? Would such a system clarify basic problems such as the respective importance of nature, nurture and culture?

ERIKSON:

I cannot answer this except as a recipient at the other end of the communication of highly fragmentary and heterogenous elements of some kind of a language. The child might be 'speaking to me' while he builds his scene, in another case the photograph of his scene will 'speak to me' half a year later, after I have studied the case history, and in another case it speaks to me only now, twelve years later, when I hear what has happened to the child since. Until I know the language, it is hard to discern nonsense.

GREY WALTER:

A last word on this—you were giving the children, as far as I can see, apart from the blocks, about as many elements as we have letters in our alphabet. Now if these are in the nature of letters, it would give them an enormous vocabulary. If, on the other hand, they are in the nature of words, the scope is much more limited. If you have only given them about twenty words, so to speak, then there is a relatively small number of things they can say. Your observations would have a different significance for us according to whether the features you observe are selected from an enormous possible range of presentation or whether the range is more limited.

FREMONT-SMITH:

Couldn't one say that the same objects are representing at one time a letter, and at another time another letter, and at another time a word, and at several times a whole sentence, and that this increases the complexity and potentiality from what, if looked at objectively and not symbolically, are a rather limited number of objects?

GREY WALTER:

Yes, I suppose you might be able to distinguish between your sexes or your children, by saying that in one case or one group of cases these objects seem to be handled as if they were letters or phonemes; but in another case, or at another age, they were handled as words, or phrases, or sentences or whole narratives. That in itself would be a very interesting way of analysing because that is the way

119

children themselves start a language. They make syllabic sounds, mere phonemes without semantic content, or with little semantic content and they build up, as we all know, an accepted language.

HUXLEY:

I think Grey Walter is begging the wrong question. This is not a language in the technical sense, but a set of sounds which are not accepted as a language. I would also think that it is not play in the strict sense. The children are constructing works of art and, of course, a work of art has to have its own vehicle of communication. If you like to call it a language in the broad sense that is all right, but in art the vehicles of communication are always multivalent learnt symbols, as Margaret Mead has said. In learning to speak, the child has to make the 'ga, ga' sound spontaneously to start with, but eventually it is learning something which is imposed upon it, a pattern that has been formalized by the culture. Here in Erikson's studies, the child is inventing something—free creation for himself, with objects that are certainly limited in their cultural implication, but with an amazing range of possibility comparable to that of an artist or a producer who is putting a play on the stage. I really do think that to try to force this business into a strict linguistic framework is begging the wrong question.

GREY WALTER:

I still maintain that this is a language in so far as they are using pre-formed symbols. There is a difference between an artist who is given a pencil and who can obviously draw as many pictures as he likes with a pencil, and one who is forced to make a *collage* from pre-formed structures.

HUXLEY:

Yes. On the other hand, these children can use this limited range of pre-formed symbols just as a poet can use words—he has only got a limited range of words but he can create poems of an amazing range of difference.

LORENZ:

The question about the noise factor in psychoanalysis in general is one that interests me deeply. Might we bring the discussion back to that? You see the question is how much randomness is superimposed on and hiding lawfulnesses? That is one very important question. When Erikson began I thought, well, how does he know that half of the children didn't just do random things without any lawfulness, without any communication function at all? And now it seems that practically none of them did.

GREY WALTER:
Well, you can tell that easily, it seems to me, and that is why I suggest a theoretical analysis. I quite agree with Huxley that one might not want to describe this behaviour as language necessarily, since this implies some use of the tongue, but this situation of Erik's is some code of communication, if you like. Now, in any code you could estimate the probable noise level very roughly, from the redundancy; how many times must a signal be repeated before its significance is certain? If the children use a highly redundant means of expression you can guess they are working on a noisy channel because it means they have got to overcome the uncertainty of communication, say by repetition. It seems to me that you have got the material there already. It would help me, personally, very much to know what the degree of redundancy is; for example, how repetitious was the expression of any particular relationship.

FREMONT-SMITH:
Redundancy might not be only due to noise.

GREY WALTER:
No, but it is one of the chief ways of guessing, when you cannot measure the noise directly.

FREMONT-SMITH:
But it is quite possible that redundancy might have an entirely different derivation from means of overcoming noise. I think this is peculiarly true of the kind of material that Erik is dealing with, where you have the repetition in child behaviour, and in child

121

play, which is far beyond any possibility of just trying to break through noise.

LORENZ:

May we come back once again to Grey Walter's question—'How do you diagnose noise in your observations?' Now, the parable of noise may be not immediately intelligible to some of us. So, let me explain it: if you record a curve of the sound waves reproduced on a gramophone record you'll find that there are a lot of irregularities superimposed upon the regular curves rendering all the single notes that go to make the music. When we hear the record played our ear is very well able to differentiate between the sound produced by the regular curves of the record and the sounds produced by its irregularity and by the shortcomings of the instrument. All the latter accidental and random waves we perceive as 'noise'. If you listen to the record longer, the noise gradually fades into the background and is not consciously perceived any more. Now, how do we make the analogous differentiation between the relevant lawfulness and the accidental noise-background in scientific observation? In the sensory data we receive both are mixed in a complete tangle. This is the question which rankled with me, because I do not know how we do it, and, of course, we do do it.

We put a fish into a tank to see its fighting movements. And now this fish—I always like to give concrete examples—rushes into one corner and slowly starts to weave to and fro with its head and none of the observers records it because everyone knows that this fish just happens, by pure chance, to be lying obliquely with one of its pectorals touching the ground and causes the weaving movements by pushing against it while continuing its permanent, rhythmical fanning movements. So an observer worth his (or her) salt knows instantly that this particular weaving of the fish's head is just 'noise'. In the next moment the fish swims free and now he suddenly starts jerking his head to and fro in another manner and instantly my student starts writing furiously to report his jerking. Now, how does one know? One knows because one has seen it before, and this is exactly where the relation between redundancy and noise, mentioned by Grey Walter, comes in. The more often the observer, or any recording machine, has recorded sets of data in which a lawfulness is mixed with random noise, the better it is able to differentiate between the two. Conversely, the more noise is contained in the sets of data, the more repetitions are necessary to be tolerably sure of the lawfulness contained in them. One knows, because one has seen it before, and recognizes it in exactly the same way as a physician recognizes some symptoms because the symptom is not a jerk in itself but is part of a syndrome. The recognition of a syndrome is slightly akin to the perception of a melody. It has a meaning, because one has seen it before. This jerk is not just a jerk, but is a very slight intentional movement, the beginning of a definite behaviour pattern. My student records it because she recognizes it. This recognition is purely perceptional, and we must confess that we do not do it by a rational act. You know how, when listening to an old gramophone for the first time, you think you hear only noise and you find it very difficult to hear the melody at all, and after a very short time you find that your perception has effected a 'retouchement' of the sensory data so that you hear only the melody at the time of playing; this suppression of noise is an achievement of Gestalt perception.

I know that when Grey Walter talks about the noise and the difficulty of eliminating it he means scientifically and mathematically abstracting from noise. In observing fish fighting, it would be very difficult to find means as rational as his, and, I must add, we have given much thought as to how we do it. I think we simply do not do it rationally, we let our perception do it, and therefore I am very interested to hear what Erikson has to say about it.

GREY WALTER:
I agree with Konrad that recognizing what is significant in a patient's condition against a background of random behaviour is a question of Gestalt perception in the sense that this means the perceiving of a whole pattern, but I suggest that the determination of what the Gestalt is, is statistical. It is a fact that a skilled person can make a significant observation of fish behaviour or of one of our electrical records, but this is achieved by a process of statistical appraisal, which need not be conscious. I suggested last time we met, in connexion with the theory of learning, that the perception of pattern *is* learning, and learning *is* perception of pattern—the two are tautologous, and the question is how particularly the psycho-analyst tunes his learning filter to admit the statistically relevant material and to exclude, or allow for, the existence of a random component in communication. The channel between the two people, the analyst and the analysand, or between Erik and his children, cannot be a perfect channel; the ideal channel has no noise level and there need be no redundancy because the communication is perfect.

123

But the ideal channel does not exist. In the technique developed by Freud and his pupils, a filter system was set up so that it is possible for the symbolic material contained in the case history or the subject's conversation or work or play to be selected against a background of conventional noise, which might in conversation be remarks as 'fine day, pity it's snowing' and so forth; a lot of polite nonsense that means nothing. Without going into details at all, the important point is that these filters are in the analyst and in the patient and the analyst's task is to match his filters to those of the subject.

The question that still remains, of course, is how he does this and then decides in his appraisal of the material, *a posteriori*, which of the signals has significance, exactly as in the observations quoted by Konrad. Konrad considers that a certain mode of behaviour is irrelevant because of certain physical facts which by a process of association he has learned reduce the significance of that behaviour. He may, for example, have discovered that in a certain situation the patient or the animal has no alternative mode of behaviour. But, in another situation, where there is less constraint, a similar mode of behaviour he *decides* is relevant. I suggest that invariably this decision is based on an acquired habit of statistical appraisal. It seems to me that, in all trained observers' experience, there is in fact a high degree of selection by scientific filtering and that Erikson has constructed an elegant filter-situation and has been making experiments with as great a significance as the experiments electrophysiologists make, where the filters are more obviously mechanical. In all such experiments the detection of a pattern depends upon the operation of statistically determined filters which are set to emphasize relevance—we EEG folk call them 'analysers' rather than analysts.

FREMONT-SMITH:

I might add one other point which bothers me a little bit—that is the complexity in the system where you have two human beings as the two objects of the communication. It becomes very hard then to define where is the end-point to which the communication is directed; the filters are actually built into the ear of the person who receives, and the person himself, who changes all the time, is very intrinsically part of the channel. We can almost say there are three or four persons at the end of the channel who are receiving his message and who are receiving it differently, and sometimes one of them receives it and sometimes another, and they also merge with one another.

GREY WALTER:
You mean that one analyst, for example, may be able to interpret or make sense of material which another analyst could not? That Erik might pass on some material which he had collected to one of his colleagues who might be able to make sense of it when Erik could not?

FREMONT-SMITH:
Yes, but also my point is that one analyst is several analysts.

GREY WALTER:
Yes, of course—or certainly a complex one—again like our electronic analysers that contain banks of filters. Just to make clear what one means by the statistical approach to such problems: in any system of observation, if you define and predict a certain pattern of behaviour, then in that system there is a finite possibility that the pattern will occur by chance—and one's duty is, either unconsciously by reason of being a clever chap, or, consciously by reason of previous training, to determine what are the possibilities of finding this pattern by chance. There is still a fundamental difficulty in all such work in deciding how likely we are to observe a certain pattern by purely chance concatenation.

The noise component in a signal is by definition unpredictable from moment to moment, but in animal behaviour, unpredictability may be quite healthy. In fact, I would add the suggestion that what a psychiatrist calls neurotic behaviour may, in some cases at least, be abnormal in so far as it *is* predictable. Of course in this problem 'predictable' has no philosophic meaning: it refers only to the limitations of the observer.

LORENZ:
Of course, the unconsciously working computer which we call Gestalt perception works on exactly the same principle as statistical deduction. It has to have the same basis of data. The likelihood of correct results is just as much dependent on the broadness of inductive basis. I always maintain that in simple observations of nature, of very complicated phenomena, it is always Gestalt perception which sees things first. This might be a personal difference, for my Gestalt perception is considerably cleverer than my inductive

125

research. And I have a very strong impression that it is the same with Erik. We are both clinical observers. Grey Walter is very highly trained in evaluating his Gestalt perception, and doing the same as us, but statistically. Most clinicians have a wonderfully trained Gestalt perception for this kind of symptoms and they are absolutely unable to tell how they do it and what is the real basis of their intuitions, as they call them. And I am, of course, convinced that the process of conscious and rational induction and that of Gestalt perception are functionally analogous.

GREY WALTER:

I'd say most of us in human neurophysiology rely very much on the Gestalt hunch—which later on we justify or discredit by making elaborate planned experiments. I think most of my colleagues would agree that most of our physiological observations or discoveries have been made by hunches—Gestalt appraisal later justified and rationalized by experiment.*

*Going over this discussion with my colleagues, the idea occurred to me that, for those of us who work in the biological domain at least, the essence of our scientific training and scientific method is: (1) to learn how to keep our hunches on the associated level, without assuming causality, either *a priori* or *a posteriori*, in this way preventing our guesses from becoming myths or superstitions: (2) learning how to design experiments to determine the direction of association, that is the causal relationships between the events which we guessed—and later proved —to be associated. Statistics have a bad name in some quarters because these two stages or planes of investigation have not always been kept distinct. In this connexion, the terms association, statistics and causality apply equally to the design of scientific experiments and to what I have suggested as the mechanism of thinking in general. For example, the development of a child, according to Erikson's schema and my translation of it (see p. 192) may be considered as the record of a person's success or failure in learning to distinguish between guessed associations and experimentally verified causal relations. Again, Erikson's observations of play are, as he says, in this sense not fully fledged experiments for, though he has established an association between history, sex, personality and play, he was not able to prove that the play behaviour was causally related to history and personality; the children may have had inborn personality traits that contributed both to their family situations and to their play, just as their inborn sex characters certainly did. It is interesting that this formal classification of method immediately reminds us of the perennial practical difficulty of assessing the respective contributions of nurture and nature to human development.

Claude Bernard, the father of physiology, specified for a 'true scientist' what we should now call an 'error-feedback system' between 'experimental theory and experimental practice'. In studying the brain specifically, of course, we have the additional difficulty that, for that organ, every experiment we make is also an experience—a distinction that our French colleagues cannot logically accept!— so that we have an additional feedback loop between subject and experimenter. None the less, what encourages me is that, as well as emphasizing the difficulties and errors and limitations of human biology, I think that discussion on these lines may help us to work out methods of study to unite our disciplines and appreciate one another's contributions.

126

LORENZ:

The German word 'Nachweis'—to prove something is a 'Nach-weis', which means the 'after-showing'—implies that you have seen it before in some other way. And I was impressed by the fact that some modern American learning-psychologists try to do without the hunch, and put the question of 'either, or'.

FREMONT-SMITH:

And become progressively more sterile!

ERIKSON:

Let me come back to these questions (in as far as I understand them) in connexion with the clinical part of our discussions. Today, I

FIG. 17

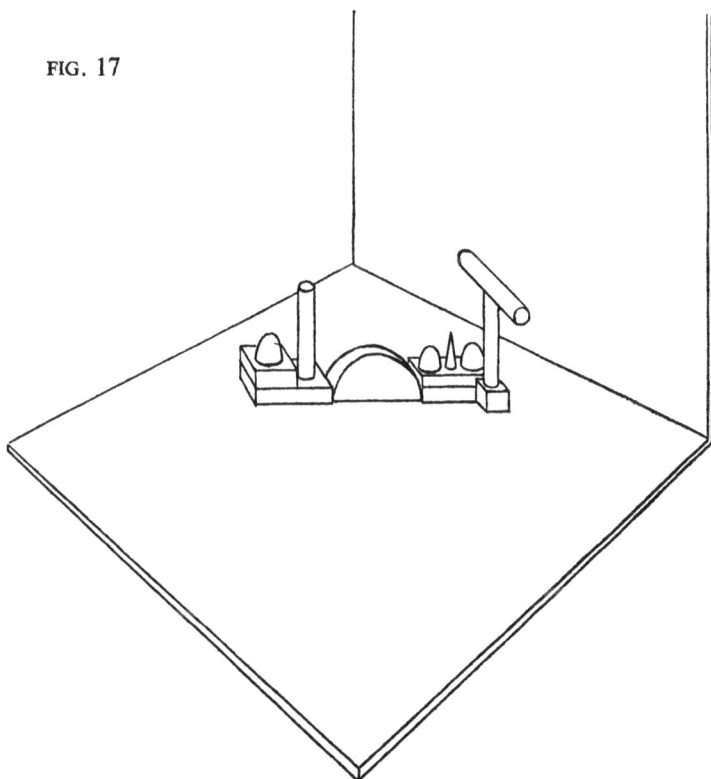

will conclude with a few examples which show how unique biographic themes will break through. Consider the construction of a boy whose mother died when he was five years old. The family had wondered at the time whether the mother could have been saved if the ambulance had come in time. His father had not discussed these circumstances with the boy and had, in fact, assumed that they had not been taken in by the child. However, our workers perceived a certain change in the boy at that time and had wondered what he knew. He remained non-committal. At age twelve, he is asked for play construction. He builds a street crossing, and explains: 'Here (in the foreground) is an ambulance driving towards that house (in the left background) where a woman is dying. As it approaches this crossroads here another car is coming out of this garage (in the right background). Ambulance and car collide. The question is

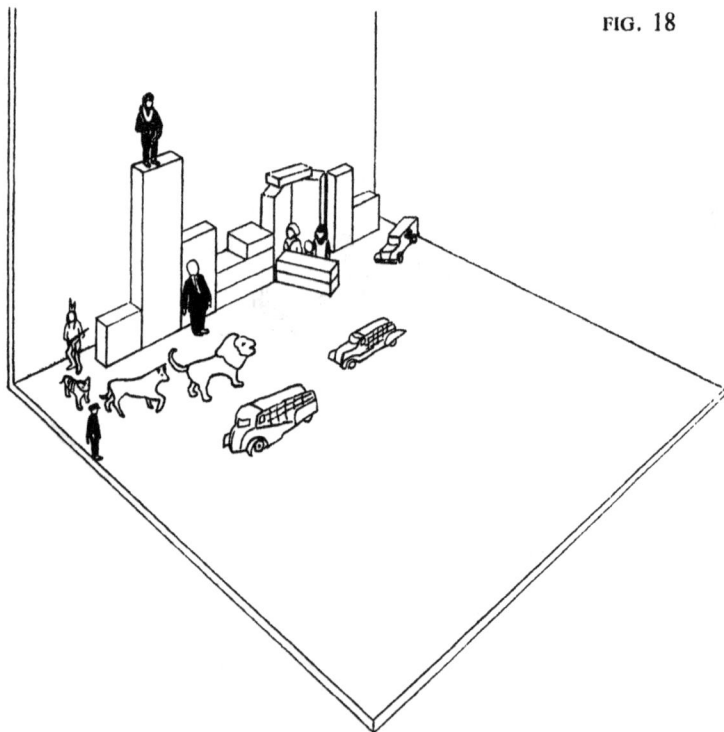

FIG. 18

128

whether the ambulance will be on time to save the woman.' I asked him 'Do you think the woman will be saved?' and he said, 'Yes, I think so'. Thus, his construction rectified circumstances which he had been supposed to be ignorant of.

Fig. 17 is one of the very few girls' constructions which consists of blocks only. It is the only one where the top is bigger than the bottom. This is a child who was born with a head deformity. This cylinder was by no means easy to balance, and she spent some time doing just that. Thus, on the one hand she wanted to show that she could balance it, while at the same time she made the top more prominent than the bottom. At the same time, the great primitivity of this construction points to an intelligence problem. I think the scene could be very well assigned to a much earlier age; there was no content to it at all.

Fig. 18 is by a child who had a congenital heart defect. She had a very much enlarged heart. It had been decided that this should not be discussed with her. She had never mentioned it, and had never been asked about it. So here again we have an example where the question is, is this biographic item which seems all-important to us, also important to this child, so important that it would appear in her play construction? Now let us see what she communicates.

She builds a tower-like structure very close to the background, as part of a kind of irregular wall. I will read the rest, from a publication.

'On the highest block stands the aviator, while below two women and two children are crowded into the small compartment of a front yard, apparently watching a procession of cars and animals. Lisa's story follows. We see in it a metaphoric representation of a moment of heart weakness—an experience which she had never mentioned 'in so many words'. The analogy between the play scene and its suggested meaning will be indicated by noting elements of a moment of heart failure in brackets following the corresponding play items.

'There is a quarrel between the mother and the nurse over money (irritability). This aviator stands high up on a tower (feeling of dangerous height). He really is not an aviator, but he thinks he is (feeling of unreality). First he feels as if his head was rotating, then that his whole body turns around and around (dizziness). He sees these animals walking by which are not really there (seeing things move about in front of eyes). Then this girl notices the dangerous situation of the aviator and calls an ambulance (awareness of attack and urge to call for help). Just as the ambulance comes around a corner, the aviator falls down from the tower (feeling of sinking and falling). The ambulance crew quickly unfolds a net; the aviator falls into it, but is bounced back up to the top of the tower (recovery). He holds onto the edge of the tower and lies down (exhaustion).'

HUXLEY:

What is the child in the foreground?

ERIKSON:

The 'older boy' doll. It was not clear whether he was left there by mistake or belonged to the construction. The girl did have an older brother.

This is a statement in the language of play regarding a most relevant experience which had not found access yet to words. However, right after the construction the girl went for a routine physical examination, where she confided to the doctor that she had strange feelings now and again. In other words, the play medium had loosened up whatever kept the communication from words.

HUXLEY:

I am coming back to the very basic point raised by Grey Walter. In anything like this—in language, in play, in art—don't you have two things involved, communication and expression. The individual expression may be forced into a more or less formal pattern, either by the limited choice of symbols which you have here, or because the pattern has been forced on you by the cultural use of a language. The children here, as far as I understand it, were essentially wanting to *express* themselves. In the background of their minds, doubtless, was the idea that this would communicate something to you, but their primary need was expression. Whereas in language, in the strict linguistic sense, the primary need is communication, which you have to learn in order to carry out. I should have thought these children are more like the artist who paints to please himself, and doesn't bother about communication.

ERIKSON:

Let me say here that I never asked any of the children whether their construction meant to them what it meant to me. I am convinced the vast majority of them would have said to me, 'Don't be silly; I just made up a scene—as you asked me to do'. Some kids might say, 'Well, aren't you pretty clever', and half acknowledge the meaning. Others might say, 'Don't be absurd'. Some might laugh,

130

some be deeply disturbed, and some be so annoyed that they wouldn't come to the next session, because why should they build movie scenes for me and then be told that 'I know something about you that you didn't know you were telling me'. But since I could not and would not confront a child with the possible meaning of his play, unless it was therapeutically indicated, it remains an open question whether self-expression contains an unconscious communication.

FREMONT-SMITH:
That that is so is emphasized by the children's preoccupation—that they were doing something for themselves, and that they had to be reminded afterwards to tell you what was exciting in it, or what it was all about.

ERIKSON:
Let me come back to the example of the boy with the plasticine balls. He knew for sure that I wanted to find out something that he had not told anybody. When he noticed I was on the right track his symptoms appeared—in other words, these hidden contents are defended against, in the individual, in varying degrees. Only patients can and must gradually accept interpretations—because they need to.

RÉMOND:
Dr. Huxley wanted to distinguish between communication and expression in order to define the content of the constructions which Mr. Erikson showed us, but I wonder whether one can in fact find any 'expression' here, at least as far as this term comprises anything intentional. Is it not just a matter of 'noise', that is to say a non-significant piece of behaviour. The child does what he does not necessarily in order to express something. He may do it just by chance. It is only after the event when he is asked what he has done that he interprets it and gives value to it. At that moment certainly expression comes in and communication as well, but did they exist before?

HUXLEY:
In these constructions that we have been seeing, although a great deal of the motivation and symbolization may have been unconscious, it seems obvious after what we have heard this morning that

131

they were expressing certain tensions, certain background or immediate discomforts and conflicts. I have been quite convinced by the demonstration. But of course the subject may afterwards give a rationalized and essentially untrue interpretation or explanation of his constructions.

The Syndrome of Identity Diffusion in Adolescents and Young Adults

ERIKSON:
I want to start with a statement made by Dr. Zazzo at one of your previous meetings. This, incidentally, is not an attempt at an advance appeasement in regard to any methodological difference we may have, but the acknowledgement of at least one common platform! He said that psychologists are perhaps wrong in looking only for the limit of intelligence, meaning at a certain age, say, the age of fourteen to eighteen. 'The age of twelve to thirteen years marks perhaps a new departure. Intelligence is nothing if it is not creative and intelligence can only be effective if it goes back to certain affective sources. Now it is perhaps during this period from fourteen to eighteen years that the human being, coming into contact with new social, human and affective realities, manages to give a deep, concrete sense to all the perceptive-intellectual mechanisms which he has acquired during the scholastic period' (Vol. I, pp. 169-70). What is said here about intelligence also applies to that accentuation of psychosexual differences which Margaret Mead spoke about. Namely, whatever has been accentuated in childhood will have to be given a deep concrete sense at this age—a sense which I call a sense of *identity*.

Now I would think that every participant in a small group like this should first characterize the kind of research experience that he is concerned with most of the time, and most intensively. I, therefore, would like to discuss clinical observations and then work toward social studies, hoping that then we can have a discussion which will combine Margaret Mead's anthropological and my clinical material in a fruitful way.

I now want to discuss one more play construction in some detail.

133

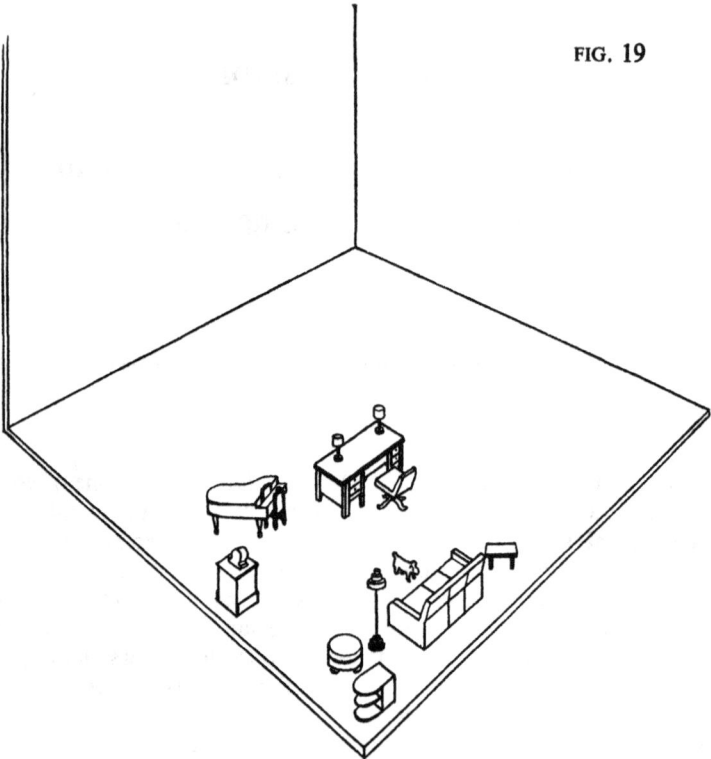

FIG. 19

The construction shown in Fig. 19 is taken from a study parallel
to the one which I undertook in Berkeley. The arrangement of table
and toys, and the instructions are the same. A girl of twelve enters.
Let me briefly account for the configurational message which I
received from her behaviour. She *walked* like a girl who 'makes
like' a boy. Yet this had an almost perfect hermaphroditic balance,
such as some girls in early puberty have. She *built* a round scene of
furniture, that is, an exquisitely feminine scene, but she built it
way out in the left forward corner, which, as I said, indicated to me
a great need for independence. Building that far out in space is often
combined with a daring of a kind which may cause the individual
to 'stick his neck out' too far. So now, we have (1) a 'boyish' style of
walking in a girlishly pretty person (2) an 'independent' location of a
'feminine' configuration. Now, within that configuration of furniture
a little *drama* took place. There was a piano and a piano chair. With
a vigorous motion the girl pushed that piano chair in, a 'unique

element' which I have noticed in only two children. It obviously connotes: 'Nobody is going to play, if I can help it'. Then the girl put a fluffy little dog in the centre of the round configuration, thus adding another typically 'feminine' element, and said 'This is it'. I asked her—'What is the most exciting thing in that scene?' and she said, 'This little dog wants to jump up on the couch and sleep'. As she said 'and sleep' she made a maternal gesture of holding and rocking a baby in her arms—a gesture such as among men only Konrad Lorenz could demonstrate. I then asked, 'What is going to happen?' and she said, 'He probably won't be able to sleep, there is too much noise'.

In addition, then, to the dualism within the configuration, you have a dramatic opposition in content, namely, the wish to rest in a soft place, and disturbing noise, and two opposed postural styles, mannish and maternal.

This girl's mother is a well-known singer. Her scene seemed to me to be a significant pointer to the fact that this girl must have been impressed, as a small child, by the fact that her mother made so much noise, and this while sitting at the piano or in conjunction with an accompanist, of whom the child may have been jealous. For their joint noise may well have drowned out the girl's own signals telling of her needs for the mother to come to her. This little scene, after so many years, says: 'If only my mother had sent the pianist away, stopped all the musical noise, and had me rest in her arms instead'. This scene, then, points to a very specific form of 'separation from the mother', one which can happen when the mother is very much there, and you can see how in a carefully arranged stimulus-situation such a basic theme simply and quickly expresses itself. A sketch of this girl's life would show that certain biographic data amount, in fact, to long-range variations, extending over many years, of the brief statement of play themes as developed in a few minutes. One of the girl's college advisers exclaimed: 'How can anybody be as dependent and as independent at the same time!'

But now let me come back to the 'message' of those few minutes. Maybe we clinicians selectively notice conflicts because it is our business to do so. On the other hand, the girl can be shown to repeat one message in a number of languages: spatial, gestural, thematic. This can be explained on the basis of Freud's repetition-compulsion, meaning that whatever experience was traumatic, i.e., rendered the individual unable to manage the quantity of excitation which stormed in on him, is repeated over and over, either through talking it out, or through redreaming it, in different variations on a theme. There is, in fact, a certain stereotyped repetition in all neurotic

135

symptoms. It came to me yesterday when we talked about communication value that such repetitiveness in a sense is like an SOS, which you repeat over and over, not only in order to get rid of inner excitation and to master the memory by repeating it actively, but also, as it were, to ask: 'Won't somebody please perceive my message and help me?'

GREY WALTER:

In such a situation, where the doctor and the patient have chosen a conventional channel to speak, and when the patient is incapable of making a really dramatic statement of conflicts or stresses—he doesn't actually come to you and say: 'For Christ's sake, help me'— then he is using for this purpose a noisy channel, and repetition may be the only means by which he can convey the information about his state and thus overcome the noise-level. Repetition may be the major feature of psychoanalytic communication because the analyst deliberately restricts his channel to the conventional means of communication—I mean in those cases where he is not using one of the more elaborate means of abreaction, such as narcoanalysis, as a means of producing material of more emphatic significance. Perhaps that is why conventional analysis is notorious for its duration and why the ultimate message seems so childishly simple in comparison with the effort.

FREMONT-SMITH:

It seems to me 'conventional' is the wrong word: the conventional means of communication is the one that the ordinary doctor or the parent uses; actually the analyst is using a variety of non-conventional means of communication which the child can send the message along.

GREY WALTER:

I mean the conventional psychiatric interview where the patient is just talking, or lying on the couch and talking, rather than hypno- or narco-analysis and so on. In those latter systems the psychiatrist is resorting to the expedient of raising the amplification, so to say. This may help but will only be confusing if the signal noise ratio is low. In a conversational or non-participatory technique repetition to the point of redundancy may be the only effective stratagem to get through the noise of a conventional channel—even when the message is really quite simple.

LORENZ:

Thomas Mann, who is a very good psychoanalyst, has realized the principle of the necessity of redundancy because of the noisiness of the channel. In his novel on Joseph (Mann, 1948) he says this explicitly where Joseph interprets the three identical dreams of the Pharaoh.

DE SAUSSURE:

You indicated as one of the characteristics of this girl that she had a conflict of dependence and independence at the same time. From the clinical point of view what characterizes her is just that these two tendencies of independence and dependence, although they are contradictory, are not conflicting in her case. She has managed to isolate these two tendencies. One of the reasons why she might have special difficulty in the formation of her identity is that through a defence mechanism she has isolated the two poles of the conflict which she has consequently never resolved.

As regards repetition-compulsion, I think that it is only in a very secondary way that repetition-compulsion acquires value as a communication. Initially, it is merely a kind of impossibility of stopping the discharge mechanism, just as in physics there is a force of inertia. The moment an unconscious charge becomes too strong it has to become apparent the whole time; so clinically what the individual is trying to do is to stop, by means of suppression or through other defence mechanisms, something which actually is striving to appear the whole time; it is only secondarily that this process is used for communication.

ERIKSON:

Yes, I merely thought that it may be valuable to take a fresh look at the repetition-compulsion from this angle. If somebody was in a train accident and then talks about it again and again, his friends find it at first interesting and then gradually boring, but they say to themselves, 'Well, he needs to do that', i.e., for the purpose of unloading traumatic excitation. But this is an accident that came from outside, and for which there are words. But I am referring here to a different situation. Let us say a little boy loses his mother when he is five. Nobody discusses it with him. He may express in any number of ways that he needs to have it discussed; these ways are not recognized and his character seems to change. Years later, the question which he wanted to ask them clearly breaks through in a play construction, and this in the same manner of a repetition of a theme on a number of levels. There may be an almost biological tendency in

137

children to try to communicate by symptomatic repetition something which they can neither say nor manage by themselves.

GREY WALTER:

It might be helpful to transfer this situation to a biological level and ask what survival-value, if any, this process has—supposing there is an inborn tendency for animals and particularly primates to repeat themselves. The IRMs that Konrad Lorenz describes are used repeatedly, are they not? Behaviour patterns appear again and again but their repetition can have very little survival-value unless it improves communication. It seems to me that there is a tendency, as Dr. de Saussure said, for the communication to be repeated by sheer momentum but that ultimately the survival-value of such a mechanism is that by repetition the signal is transmitted more accurately. The two are not incompatible by any means; the mechanism may be an inborn individual character, but the advantage may depend on social gain in clarity when there are many other things going on. It might be interesting to know from the biological standpoint to what extent the tendency to repeated behaviour patterns has, in fact, a high survival-value.

LORENZ:

I think that it is permissible to identify the compulsive repetition of which Erikson is talking with the repetition of instinctive activity in normal animals. Yet the question whether this repetition is adaptive, has a survival value or not, is something which has very strongly occupied me already, because I am subject personally to very strong compulsion to repetition of traumatizing experiences in which I misbehave, in which I fail to behave in the manner I like to remember myself having behaved—in other words, in situations where I have made a fool of myself. In such cases I have to go through and through this experience again, re-enacting the scene and saying the things I ought to have said to the chap.

HUXLEY:

So that there are really two grades, aren't there? The first is the basic impulse to perform a certain type of action as a result of the conflict; and the second the later stereotyping of it either individually or in evolution, as a means of communication. Displacement activities, for example, may be *expressions* in origin, serving to get rid of excess tension, while later on they become a means of communication.

138

BOWLBY:
I find Konrad's point an interesting one because what has always puzzled me is this: people find it much easier to get over a traumatic situation if they can communicate about it to others. Erik has already given the example of the way in which, after an accident, we bore all our friends by describing it again and again. In some way the mere expression of it, particularly the repetition of it to people we like, with whom we have a particular bond, enables us to get over it, to adapt to it and forget it. Now, the striking thing about neurotic patients is that they cannot do this in respect of some important event or sequence of events. It looks as though what happens is not that this mechanism, which has a healing and survival-value as Konrad described, persists too long and becomes patho-logical, but that it fails to start at all. It then requires a new person to enable the healing process to start and achieve its proper end.

If we consider the child whose mother died and who was never able to discuss that event, from clinical experience we agree that, had he been able to discuss and adapt to the event in the period immediately following, this healing process would have been completed efficiently. As it was, since there was no one with whom he could communicate, this didn't occur at the time and the healing process ceased. It wasn't until a new situation arose—a situation of communication—that the healing process began again. I would emphasize strongly the com-municative significance of the play session which Erik had with these children. The fact that Erik is there as a human being de-termines the situation—and I would expect that the precise com-munications which these children made were very dependent on their perception of Erik as a human being.

DE SAUSSURE:
If one gives to a hypnotized person a post-hypnotic order which he cannot completely carry out, he repeats it or repeats something which is intermediate. For example in one of the cases quoted by Moll (1889) in his work on hypnosis, he gave the order to a very timid girl to stretch out her hand to him as soon as she woke up. The moment she stretched out her hand she began to tremble and from that moment every time she wanted to stretch out her hand she began to tremble without being able to shake hands. Here we see behaviour which is repeated because it has not been able to be com-pletely expressed. We also note that there has been no correction; this girl has not improved her behaviour after x times; she does not shake hands any better. On the other hand, as soon as Moll had

hypnotized her again and had made a stronger suggestion she became capable of giving her hand without trembling.

We see that this repetition is much more an expression than a
communication; if there were communication there would be improvement.

In neurotic situations the phenomena are much more complex.
There are at the same time elements of repetition-compulsion (as
in post-hypnotic cases) and elements of communication. It is
owing to the latter that behaviour improves and the general situation
changes.

The example quoted by Erikson of this child who was never able
to speak of the death of his mother is precisely an example of un-
finished discharge because the discharge should have come from
outside, which creates a much more complicated situation.

The example quoted by Lorenz about his own behaviour, which
forced him to repeat a certain reaction a certain number of times,
was different because the behaviour came from him whereas in the
case of the child the incitement to discharge came from outside.
It is possible, therefore, that favourable circumstances would permit
him suddenly to discharge his emotion and an improvement would
follow. It is for this reason, too, that the communication element is
much stronger in a neurotic situation than in an experimental
situation, for example.

ERIKSON:

We come here to a generalization which is important to our
further discussion, namely, the containment of the mere discharge
in a workable communication. The girl of twelve could push in the
piano chair in the play scene; in other words, she had the medium
and the capacity to do symbolically what she would have done in
reality when she was a child—if she had not been a child. Because of
the long-drawn-out childhood in human beings, the traumatization
by events in which we are unable to communicate simply because
we are children, i.e., are not listened to, or have no means of communicating, is of a specific quality. I would say that the mere humili-
ation of having been a child is one of the most basic facts of human
existence.

It so happens that my quotation from Shaw's autobiographic notes
(Erikson, in press) contain an item which I call 'the noise-maker',
which will provide a fitting transition to my next point. When Shaw
was 70, he was asked to write a preface to five novels which he had
written in his early twenties in five years, writing five pages each

day. He did this compulsive feat during a period which I will later call a psychosocial moratorium. He was a clerk in an Irish merchandizing house and he was not unsuccessful by any means, but he felt not like himself in this situation. He left Ireland, went to England, and he said he did not intimately associate with members of his own age group for something like seven years. You find such self-imposed psychological moratoria in the life of quite a number of outstanding people. So when he was a famous man then it was decided to publish those five novels, and he wrote a preface to them. Of course, he ended up by saying—for heaven's sake don't bother to read those five novels but listen to my description of what kind of a human being I was when I wrote them. He wrote one of the sharpest autobiographical statements which I have ever read. It is not known as a major psychological work simply because Shaw had the additional compulsion to make everything seem funny. At the end of this autobiography he says in regard to his identity as an actor on the stage of life, 'in this, I succeeded only too well', a statement of integrity which admits that some are forced by their very identity formation into successes which feel just a little too good.

Among the many elements that Shaw described in his own development is the identity of the music critic—his first identity as a writer, the novels having failed him as he failed them. He describes how, when he was a child, he was exposed to an oceanic assault of music making; his sisters and uncles and cousins played trombones, violincellos and harps and tambourines—and, most of all, his mother sang! During his psychosocial moratorium (which, as I said, I will define later) he taught himself the piano and he did this with the utmost of noise that he could manage. He says 'When I look back on all the banging, whistling, roaring and growling inflicted on nervous neighbours during this process of education, I am consumed with useless remorse. . . . I used to drive (my mother) nearly crazy by my favourite selections from Wagner . . . which seemed horribly discordant at that. She never complained at the time, but confessed it after we separated, and said that she had sometimes gone off to cry. If I had committed a murder I do not think it would trouble my conscience very much; but this I cannot bear to think of.' If you will permit an interpretation which Shaw does not propose himself, he did not, as it were, cancel out the trauma of having been invaded and assaulted with musical noise as a child, he turned it around and did it to other people, calling it his education. Only later, at a time when he had made enough noise to abreact, as we would say, did he become aware of the aggressive nature of his musical self-education. But now he compromised by becoming somebody who

141

writes about the musical noise other people make, and this led him closer to his identity as a writer, and sublimated his aggression in criticism. The name he chose as a music critic, incidentally, was Corno di Bassetto. The few people who know it, know that it was the meekest musical instrument in existence. He said 'not even the devil could have made it sparkle'. You see the strange way in which people can manage their lives if their culture gives them leeway to do so, and if they are gifted in utilizing this leeway. As Corno di Bassetto, he became a music critic who was in no way meek, in fact, he said, 'I cannot deny Bassetto was occasionally vulgar; but that does not matter if he makes you laugh. Vulgarity is a necessary part of a complete author's equipment.'

In Shaw was a man of genius, which includes the gift of finding his identity as he imposes it on the world. One might say that his autobiography was part of his professional work, he lived a professional autobiography. This is, of course, one extreme of identity formation, if one of the most instructive ones. Shaw says about his youth, 'everyone is ill at ease until he has found his natural place, whether it be above or below his birthplace', but then being Shaw, he has to add 'This finding of one's place may be made very puzzling by the fact that there is no place in ordinary society for extraordinary individuals'. How many people feel they are extraordinary even if they neither have the gift of Shaw to impose his identity on his neighbours, nor live in a period in which enough space is given for such special realization of themselves? We seem to be living at a time when, in many areas of the world, the choices are very much reduced and the need for conformity very much increased.

But this is what I would like to end up with tomorrow and not what I would like to start with. So now I would like to finish this morning with a very general statement as to what I consider identity to be, and with a brief example of what a transitory failure in identity formation would look like. To find one's identity in late adolescence means to find an orientation toward one's self and others in which one feels most oneself where one has come to mean most to others, i.e., to those others who are closest. This is by necessity a statement of relativity, because as we grow we move within a changing and expanding group of people. We select as we are selected and this interchange must lead at the end of adolescence to a feeling that what one means to others, and what one feels one is, largely coincide. You might also say that the sense of identity is a sense of inner continuity and sameness in development, in that what one was made to expect as a child, and what one can anticipate that one will be, coincides with what one is. We will go into all of this in detail later—

142

here I would just like to emphasize the sometimes fatal, sometimes happy relativity of it all.

A happy aspect is what I would refer to as mutual recognition. I have a small collection of interviews which I had in one great university with the most gifted batch of doctoral students. With great regularity during their formative years, one teacher or aunt or friend of the family became very important, partially because the student became very important to that individual, and a mutual recognition took place which I think is very important for finding one's self as a young individual. Obviously, this can be with a master to whom one is an apprentice, with an older friend who wishes to be selected as a guide, or some neighbour, relative or friend who says the right thing at the right time. For this recognition to occur the individual needs three things: he needs to be free enough from his past problems to be able to choose the right person or the group of people, who have a recognition in store. Then there must be people in existence who are looking for just the kind of young person he is. Finally, it needs certain cultural circumstances which favour the two meeting.

Identity diffusion is something that which occurs when this is not possible, at the right time and in a certain proper dosage. Identity diffusion is a syndrome that many young people have in common, although its forms are seen as sicknesses or bad habits with a variety of causes. If people with identity diffusion are found in a certain acute bewilderment, they may be suspected of being schizophrenic. If they happen to appropriate a car—because to drive around in a car gives them the feeling they are somebody—they become delinquents, and if they happen to cross a State line, maybe Federal offenders. If they use drugs to feel like whole people, they are on the way to addiction. In all of this it is important to know that whatever the inner dynamics, there is a relatively autonomous factor common to youth, namely, that whatever the representatives of society will tell a young person he is, he is more apt to become. I mean here something which I believe is in a way analogous to imprinting in the sense that the young individual is ready to respond selectively, even as his environment is (or should be) ready to recognize him as such and such, and to offer him a series of mutual responses through which he would find out what, within the roles of his culture, he can make of himself as he is. I say this, because eventually we should come out with a unified theory which includes all of childhood or pre-adulthood, from the mutuality with the mother in babyhood, to that with a segment of society in late adolescence.

Let me now turn to therapeutic material, and with it to my home

143

ground as observer. The role of the therapeutic observer is one that is only now being studied systematically, in the sense that he should learn to understand better what kind of an instrument he is, what kind of instrument he becomes as he works with patients, day after day. When I read the reports of your previous meetings, I was flooded with envy as I conceived of you as people who have time to arrange experiments, to observe, to think, to converse, during all those many, many hours which we spend with individual patients. And yet one should hope that even in such individual observation one would become an instrument that recognizes and conceptualizes some kind of regularity. Let me discuss briefly a number of pitfalls in therapeutic observation, because the recognition of its 'equations' circumscribes the use of an instrument in at least one relevant way. Anybody who is forced by human misery to play, and tempted to overplay, his role as a helper and as a systematizer, will by necessity come to short circuits in his own attitude toward people and the world in general. We therapeutic observers have a contract with the material under observation. The contract says that through observation we hope to help the patient back into life in an improved condition. We cannot ask him any question, even if it is based on an ever so good hunch, out of mere theoretical interest, if the question is a violation of the contract, although at times the very contract will oblige us to make him feel worse, before we can make him feel better. However, we can never plan experiments for the purpose of finding out what does not work; we must always unequivocally support the therapeutic process: thus each insight derived from the understanding of failure is bought at the expense of a much more personal failure than is true in dealings with other material. Now this particular contract certainly, as Grey Walter would say, defines the 'band' of our receptivity.

[Mr. Erikson then presented an example of an episode of severe identity diffusion in a young man of about twenty-two who was preparing to do missionary work. He discussed the patient's history, emphasizing those images in the family history which provided the growing child and youth with an inventory of identity fragments too irreconcilable to be integrated during his identity crisis.

(1) the family's migration from rural Minnesota to industrial-urban Pittsburgh; the parents' nostalgic attachment to Minnesota and the family's visits there (the pure 'North country', agrarian, ethnically and religiously homogeneous, 'old country' tradition;

144

the smoky city, ethnic 'melting pot', emphasis on success and progress).

(2) the mother's attitude toward babies and children of varying ages, her loving trust in smaller children and her concern and despair in the face of certain tensions connected with the growing-up of an impetuous boy (association of 'back home' in history and geography and early childhood in life-history).

(3) the boy's vigorous and impatient, yet sensitive temperament, and its contrast with the mother's image of a small child.

(4) early conflicts between voracious dependence (wish to get everything any time, and without end) and need to get away from mother (association of having hurt mother by being vigorously independent and having forfeited the happiness of early childhood —of the North country—of the homogeneous past).

(5) his early conflict between fear of and identification with the city-bred, ruder, 'lower', and ethnically more mixed children of the neighbourhood, of whom his family seemed to disapprove; the phallic-aggressive orientation of the 'education' bestowed by certain boy leaders on the neighbourhood children; their bragging about sexual freedom, and the occasional free discussion of incest; delinquencies related to automobiles; abortive 'gangs'.

(6) the boy's discovery of the saxophone as an instrument permitting both loud and tender expression, and as a 'social tool', permitting both distance from and belongingness to a certain high-school 'crowd'. His family's mistrust of that crowd and their limited approval of that magic instrument, the saxophone.]

Mr. Erikson continued: Those who like to play jazz not only make concerted aphonic noise, but also develop a particular language, particular nicknames, a proudly deviant subculture which gives many an individual—especially if one does not fit in anywhere else—a home, as it were, at any rate a transitory one. These people 'recognized' in our patient a 'hepcat' and he became, and still is today, a very good saxophone player. Those of you who know the American novel *From Here to Eternity* will remember the touching and tragic case of a young soldier, to whom his trumpet had become an essential extension of himself, an 'oral outlet', a tool to express perfection, and a bond with other people, and the vehicle of a private religion which helped him to overcome murderous identifications—until society deprived him of it.

[Mr. Erikson then discussed the patient's relationship to his father, who, as a soil conservationist and plant pathologist, had found a quiet and constructive place in a bustling and competitive community. He continued to demonstrate inter-relationships between:

(1) the boy's association of his father's love for plants (that which grows without passion or malice) and his mother's for babies (who need you more than they want to leave you) both of which left him with the feeling of being too loud, too locomotor, too 'criminal'. The boy's intense jealousy of father's and mother's objects of care.

(2) the patient's attempt, in late adolescence, to follow his father into his profession, a sudden break-through of bewildering, aggressive impulses, and the attempt to over-compensate these by a sudden turn to missionary work—work which would combine rebellious flight from home and locomotor search for another land with the ascetic task of becoming paternal-maternal himself in the role of saving 'savage' souls. It thus would also express what real trust he *had* experienced and an almost excessive acknowledgement of his parents' love.

(3) the conflicting roles in the schooling of missionaries: all proving equally 'available' to him—the 'practical missionary' because of his vigorous devotion; the 'studious teacher' because of his outstanding gift for Asiatic languages; the 'religious advertising man', because of a certain histrionic toughness, originally associated with jazz.

(4) certain irreconcilable elements in the patient's psychosexual and psychosocial development.

(5) available diagnoses for such a disturbance.]

Mr. Erikson continued: I hope that it is quite clear that I do not for a moment doubt that the diagnosis is important; that an identity diffusion of a severely neurotic type will have to be treated differently from a paranoid or psychopathic one. Nevertheless, what I pointed out in very rough outline gives the *psychosocial* dimension of the crisis which left this individual in an inescapable dilemma.

FREMONT-SMITH:
Was it a sudden break?

ERIKSON:
It was a break that took weeks to develop. At the time he wrote to a friend 'The air here is bad, this is only half air, the rest is heavy

exhaust and virulent gases that hang like a shroud over the city and sicken your lungs, until you feel like the half air had made you half alive'. Well, such a statement can be a paranoid reference to a poisoning environment; it can be an exaggerated form of the well-known complaint concerning 'smog', and yet I would say it is also the language of sensitive young people who thus express their being suffocated by conflicting identifications. At any rate the young missionary tried to pray by staying in church all night and finally became aware of the fact that his suffering was somehow outside of his prayers. He says 'It is a curse which has personal meaning and has come from nowhere' and finally, he wrote to a friend 'It seems to me that only a complete collapse can force me to re-examine my life'. This is not an empty phrase. A certain kind of collapse at this age can be semi-intentional. Some young people think themselves deeper into the collapse because they feel that only on the rock bottom, as it were, can they find a true moratorium and a new beginning.

LORENZ:
They do their utmost to dissolve, like the chrysalis of the butterfly which dissolves almost absolutely before re-formation.

HUXLEY:
Isn't it like shock treatment in that shock destroys some neurophysiological structuring and gives the patient the opportunity to rebuild a new structure, a new pattern?

ERIKSON:
It so happened that the friend, who had been the recipient of the letters I mentioned, engaged with him in an impressive theological correspondence as to where the point is when it would be almost a sin to try and solve a conflict as a religious one, challenging God to do a miracle for the individual, while the love of God somewhere presupposes the capacity to believe in some other human being, who may have the means of help. It was in this mood that he sought psychiatric treatment.

If one is called upon to help a man who has found his identity but suffers from inhibitions or anxieties, the situation is different. Let me make it clear that there are neurotic inhibitions or symptoms which go together with a reasonably good identity formation. In this case, one only wants to resolve inhibitions and phobias which are leftovers from the past kept alive by the present. Here a psychosocial moratorium, an additional identity formation is not called

147

for. Now, in America 'classical' neuroses become rare, except in certain areas. In Pittsburgh I hear much about American families who still have ten or eleven children, with grandparents who still speak only Polish or Czech—miners' families and steelworkers' families. There, old forms of neurosis are relatively more prevalent. Otherwise the so-called classical cases are disappearing in America for the simple reason that in America getting something like a solid identity formation is becoming even harder than in some other parts of the world. However, if I may misquote Konrad Lorenz— in this case the exception of today may well be the rule of tomorrow, which means that what is now identity disturbance in particular individuals, and on a large scale in America, may well enter other areas as industrialization progresses.

In the kind of patients that I am speaking of, there are experiences during the day, and dreams at night, which clearly show the need of the patients to see themselves reflected in a friendly, and, as it were, consistent, unharmed, and unhurried face. The patient mentioned had a dream in which he saw a person whose face was surrounded by white hair (like the therapist's) travel in a horse and buggy (such as his grandfather had used) through the Minnesota countryside. The face of that person turned into a horrible Medusa-like mask, and he was not sure it was not his mother. In this dream we can see the present (therapy) condensed with the most trustworthy past (the 'old-fashioned' grandfather, now dead) and the mother's face. That face, of course, had left an 'imprint' of the earliest conflict between basic trust (hope, love) and mistrust (Medusa) in early childhood. The dream illustrates how in the identity crisis (at the end of childhood) the earliest conflicts may have to be resolved once more. I may add that the image of the homogeneous grandparent is waning in America, yet in many families the last integrated personality roles for a number of generations were those of early settlers of pre-industrial times, or maybe early industrial captains, managers or workers. The children, when they took their hand or made them read stories of a homogeneous life, felt in them something which is very hard at this moment for many children to gain from their parents. That is especially true where mothers do not trust themselves, in either representing tradition or their own tastes or even the public's changing tastes, and orient themselves by what the experts say in magazines. The trouble is, of course, that tradition cannot change as fast as the experts' opinions, so that all of this is bewildering for children.

In the treatment of such a patient, then, I would combine an attempt to define the patient's present social experiences as clearly as possible, with the discussion of 'transference' phenomena, and that of corresponding infantile conflicts. This, of course, means that the therapist has to concern himself with social facts. It also means that rather disturbed young persons in many cases can regain or maintain a much greater ability to work and to judge social situations than they would under a prolonged vacation from work life when, especially at this age, they are in danger of making the role of being a patient the basis of their identity. This is a general danger in America right now—to be a patient under psychoanalysis in some circles is a perfectly good full-time occupation, and provides status in itself. We experts now have to re-define our relationship to the culture in which we live. But this, too, means we have to acquire knowledge of psychosocial processes.

In missionary school, the patient we have been discussing had been an outstanding student of Chinese. During treatment he made use of the particular American moratorium which permits, and in fact encourages, young people of any class to be workmen for a while. Here he learned that any occupation has its own code and its own restrictions and limitations. Young people often think that it is in occupations far away from their parents, that the happy people live, the consistent and the honest people. It is often a part of the symptom of identity diffusion that everybody else, such as the people in Paris, the people in the country, or wherever one isn't, seem to be the happy and the decent people. They are the ones with a free and healthy sexuality, who love their work and are free of anxiety. It is, therefore, good for such patients to learn to know work situations, but, of course, they can at first tolerate work situations only if they do not mean continuation of their own careers, and thus long-range commitments. When my patient, for the first time, really enjoyed his work in a steel mill, he said aloud to himself—'My God, this is as good as studying Chinese!' This is a strange statement, but maybe you will understand that to me, it was a good sign, for he had realized that any number of work methods carry their own satis-faction within them, and while at this moment he would not have wanted to go back to Chinese, at any rate he had accepted work as such as an important part of himself.

GREY WALTER:
Do these Medusa dreams have any primary sexual significance?

ERIKSON:
I am sure they do, as a gaping 'void', a vacuum, the 'inner space' of the female. The Medusa's face with open mouth and surrounded by hair in the form of snakes was thus interpreted by Freud.

GREY WALTER:

I was surprised that your interpretation was mainly cultural. I should have thought there were so many personal symbols there as well, which could be equally important for the communication aspect of this therapeutic experience.

ERIKSON:

I speak of the cultural aspects here because we are discussing identity formation, not therapy or communication as such. My point is that such dreams contain the negative mother image of early childhood, i.e., they contain in condensed form all the moments when the mother felt strange, dangerous, or unhappy. In other words, while as a late product they are symbolic of the sexual horror of femininity, the facelessness also represents a concentrate of that typical early experience, when the mother becomes a frightening stranger. What I hope to indicate here is the way in which such early mistrust can continue through childhood and become embedded in those identity problems which reach a crisis in late adolescence.

BOWLBY:

My own approach to dreams of this kind, especially if they occur early in the treatment, would be to see to what extent I could determine the patient's feelings towards me from the material in the dream. The kind of way I would approach it would be: to what extent is he seeing me as a damaged and damaging mother? Or alternatively, to what extent is he seeing me as an amiable and protective grandfather? It would appear to me that these are at least possibilities alternating in his mind. The other aspect of it, to which I would give attention, would be the possibility, or perhaps likelihood, that the mother is not merely a mother who might be dangerous to him. He is dangerous to the mother also, because when he did things she didn't like, she cried. Therefore, he was always damaging her and, no doubt, she conveyed that to him in rather effective and implicit ways. My own preoccupation in such a situation with a patient would be to ask myself to what extent is he afraid of hurting me in the present treatment situation, and how much guilt and anxiety he is experiencing in the treatment vis-à-vis myself in the here and now.

ERIKSON:

I am completely in agreement. I reported the cultural aspect here as an introduction to our theme of 'the psychosocial development of the child'. Therapeutically, I would deal with it by a combination of what you have just said and what I said earlier. I would call the culture difference into the therapeutic interpretation, explaining, for example, the grandfather's actual historical position and his more homogeneous background. I also would try to objectify the mother's suffering for him, to clarify her position in her own life, and his position in her life, and so on. I would think that it is this combination which is called for, for the mere question (which I would, indeed, bring up with such patients) 'Did you feel that you could, or would, or did damage me?' can at times increase the magic danger for him, and, as it were, verify the infantile-paranoid position that if anything happens to a significant emotional partner, he must have caused it.

Now, I would like to list quickly the particular components of the syndrome called *identity diffusion*, whether it has a paranoid or other kind of flavour. May I say that Professor Huxley suggests we should call it dispersion and not diffusion, which you may want to discuss.

So if we now may turn from extreme (if transient) pathology back towards the universal elements in this 'normative crisis': I would say that every young person has these feelings at one time or another, and they are implicit in many things young people do. I in no way assume they must be pathological. I have already mentioned a *sense of time diffusion*, namely, a morbidly changed attitude toward the flow of time, toward past and present. To some extent this is an aspect of adolescence, elaborated by the specific conditions of adolescence in given cultures. In Germany when the preoccupation with ruins was a romantic hobby, young people would be preoccupied in their poems with ruins and with the beauty of the dead past. Each item that I will mention now I consider a possible aspect of extreme pathology; more often one of transitory pathology, and most generally one of adolescent imagery, which in various countries is variously connotated.

A second item is *identity consciousness*—that means an extreme form of self-consciousness. You are constantly conscious of your own appearance and with your impression on others. This is something which in the normal adolescent is a transitory matter, and in some people persists, and this not only in pathological cases but also in many creative people, which may account for a certain vanity of some creative people, a preoccupation with their own biography.

Another very important aspect is *negative identity*. The negative identity would comprise everything which a young person has learned he should *not* become. Some young people, when they feel that what they have been equipped with for life is not sufficient to create a positive identity, quite suddenly 'decide' on a negative one.

151

For example, a young person can become a borderline psychotic or an addict or a delinquent, or he may suddenly, in rather a spectacular way, become something which his parents had no idea they were indirectly fostering throughout his early life.

Young people sometimes 'choose' to become patients, because that is the only thing that they can become under the circumstances considering what they have brought along with them and what the world offers them. This, of course, can become a kind of pathological youth movement. You have groups of addicts in the large cities, you have groups of homosexuals often with little real and lasting homosexuality being developed in individuals. It is more a way of life with these young people, who feel that they are 'somebody', because at least the homosexuals will say that they belong. It gives them, at least for a period, more of an identity than they would have at home or at work, or in college, where they may feel that everything that is said to them excludes their kind from the potentialities of their culture. There is at the moment, apparently, a world-wide problem of young people looking for identity in strangely clad gangs. You may remember that in Los Angeles and in Southern California we have the 'zoot-suiters'; those are young boys with a particularly large, flat hat and with outfits that are very dandy-like. This is a tendency which has gone round the whole world, with similar names even. In Israel I met a psychiatrist from South Africa, who told me about a development among the Negroes in South Africa, and said, 'We call them the zootsies'. I think the anthropologists would call it 'culture diffusion!' Then you may have heard that in Russia there are complaints about gangs of young men in strange dress.

HUXLEY:
In London their counterparts are the teddy-boys, who dress in Edwardian style.

ERIKSON:
I emphasize this merely because this negative identity can be supported by a uniform which makes one something that does not fit the culture—it fits in the Edwardian era, or it fits into Mexico rather than into America, or into America rather than Russia, and so on. Here we would find a connexion with the enormous appeal of 'positive' youth movements in uniform who are idealistic but revolutionary.

Then I have discussed already *work paralysis*, the inability to work or unwillingness to work and the loss of that particular pleasure of work completion which this boy expressed by saying, 'The steel mill is almost as good as Chinese'.

Then there is the sense of *bisexual diffusion*. Such young people have states in which they do not feel quite clearly as members of one sex or the other, which of course very much makes them possible victims of the way of life of homosexuals or of an ascetic turning away from sexuality, with dramatic breakthroughs of impulses.

There is also *authority diffusion*, which means that they can neither simply obey nor give orders. Any situation of rivalry and competition, any situation of hierarchy of authority makes them feel panicky. And, finally, there is *ideological diffusion*, which has already been mentioned.

Now, to turn to the positive side. Each one of these items is a potential danger, I would think, at one time or another for an adolescent. However, there is in any working social structure a complete set of complementary institutions which help the individual to alleviate all of these aspects of identity diffusion. Ideological movements of great variety give an answer to all of these problems such as giving *time perspective* to the individual by interpreting what he is doing and what his society is doing in a particular way so that, at least for a while, he will know where he is and where he is going; by giving him a *self-certainty*, in regard to what he is, permitting him a certain amount of role experimentation, say, as a student or an apprentice, or a member of a fraternity or a youth group, by permitting him occupational choices that he can experiment with until he can choose a final one.

TANNER:

I wonder if you examined, with this sort of thing in mind, people who have been expatriated either forcibly or from their own choice? At the end of the war, I had to do with the psychiatric rehabilitation of returning prisoners of war, and they had a very recognizable syndrome. It was partly depression; but what you are saying about dispersion of identity seems now very relevant to the symptoms that they were having. The one thing which impressed itself on us very much during this rehabilitation, was that these 'neurotic' POW's were not constitutionally predisposed or 'proper' neurotics, but simply people who had been isolated from their culture, and had developed queer ideas of their culture during this period of isolation. When they came back, one of the things which had a great effect on rehabilitating them was a system we started of sending them out to work on the work bench with other people in the local community;

they tried four or five different sorts of work each. This was probably the most effective single measure.

HARGREAVES:
It is interesting that in the British programme for the rehabilitation of repatriated prisoners of war the term 'job rehearsal' was developed to cover this phenomenon.

HUXLEY:
Isn't it really role-rehearsal, not merely job-rehearsal?

TANNER:
If you put it as role-rehearsal, perhaps I should say that the other chief therapeutic thing was learning how to dance with the nurses!

ERIKSON:
This remark is a very fitting one. During the war I worked in a rehabilitation clinic and I would not be surprised (it's so hard to know these things about oneself) if it was not the one decisive experience which made me take the identity problem seriously. I saw some very disturbed men there, who had broken down because of long isolation and most of all because of the long preoccupation with work patterns that were not their own and could not be related to anything they had learned. To play the role of the soldier 24 hours a day is pretty hard for the majority of Americans. This has to do with the particular identity which is prepared in American youth, namely, the belief that you live for your chance; there is what amounts to a deification of The Chance in American life (your time will come —the right thing will come along—don't let anybody make a sucker out of you—don't let anybody fence you in, etc.). Under conditions of war and of industrial organization such beliefs pose a very difficult identity problem.

* * *

PIAGET:
I have been most interested by the remarks made by Mr. Erikson before he described the case at the end of the morning. He made a general observation about the way that family experiences and, particularly, the satisfactions or the difficulties of the child in relation to his mother and father later condition his successive experiences, and in particular his adaptation to society. This problem seems to me to raise questions as regards the process itself, that is as regards the explanation of this continuity, and I should like to put one

154

or two questions to Mr. Erikson especially from these two points of view. The first of these problems is the analogy with intelligence and cognitive processes in general in which we find also continuities of this kind. Then the second problem is the explanation of this continuity itself.

First, I would like to say a few words about the analogies with intelligence. When we study the development of cognitive functions, sensori-motor development, the development of perceptions and of patterns of intelligence, we continually find that early experiences or experiences from far back can equally have an importance throughout life and can orient research and orient solutions in many cases. I am not, of course, speaking of the conscious applications of previous methods or previous solutions to new problems; on the contrary, I am speaking of unconscious transfers and unconscious generalizations, and on this plane it seems to me that there is a possible comparison with the continuity of affective life. For example, on the sensori-motor level the infant makes all kinds of experiments with his hands which will play a considerable part in the organization of space, in causality, etc. and these initial experiments can explain therefore, by unconscious analogies certain choices between intellectual solutions which will occur later. But it is not only a question of general phenomena; even in the biography of individuals and in the differences between individuals we find these kinds of continuity between old situations and present situations, and this can occur at any age. If I might take an example from my own biography to help you understand what I want to say: before I became involved in psychology, I dealt with zoology, I dealt with terrestrial molluscs, that is to say with problems which do not seem to have any connexion with psychology. However, there are connexions; there is the fundamental problem of the relations between the hereditary structure and the environment, the problem of genotypes and phenotypes that we were speaking of last year and which we find now come to the fore in psychology. But when I began considering how I approached a psychological problem, and especially during discussions with colleagues, seeing that our points of view and starting points were different, I often found that there was an unconscious continuity and that without wishing to do so I thought as I had thought formerly, that the same way of posing problems keeps coming back. This dates from an education very far back and of which frequently one is not conscious. It is because of these least conscious things that very frequently we put questions in a way which is incomprehensible to our partners or contradictors. So it seems, and this is my first point, that there are fundamental analogies between this continuity of old experiences and of present situations from the affective and cognitive points of view. One finds parallel processes in both fields.

Now I come to my second problem, which is that of interpretation. There are two fundamental interpretations of continuity which is both affective and intellectual: that which I will call static interpretation and that which I will call dynamic interpretation. Static interpretation consists in saying that the individual clings to old conflicts. These old conflicts are recorded somewhere in the form of latent conflicts to which are attached memories and unconscious representations. Then throughout life, and especially at the moment of his moulding as an adolescent and at the beginning of adult work, the individual without knowing it assimilates to the present a past which has been preserved entire. It is the solution calling for this preservation of the past just as it stands which I will call the static solution.

Secondly, there can be a dynamic solution, that is to say that the past can be preserved, not in the form of conflicts buried in the unconscious, or of memories or representations buried in the unconscious, but in the form of what I will call action patterns and reaction patterns which are more like habit than memory. That is to say, one gets into the habit of reacting in a certain way, one reacts first in a certain way towards one's family, and reacts again in the same way in analogous situations, so that here is something which is more comparable to continuity in the cognitive field, where obviously it is not the unconscious memory of former situations which acts on the present, but attitudes of mind, modes of reactions, which are preserved and applied to new situations. In the second interpretation there would not be preservation of the former conflict, but the individual would continue to re-create the same conflicts. He would live through situations which are reproduced, which are re-created, without there being necessarily conservation, which seems to me personally to be somewhat difficult to explain in the unconscious. In the same way from the cognitive point of view he would continually adapt former solutions to present problems simply through the continuity of reaction patterns and not by conservation of anything.

HUXLEY:
Isn't there a third possibility which is like the second, but in which you regard the internal situation, the conflict, the method of reacting, as itself a psychological organ capable of development and change? The change in this case is analogous to maturation but not entirely automatic and intrinsic; it is related to external changes,

so that you could have intrinsic organs for dealing with conflict themselves changing in the course of time. That is how conflicts can get resolved, isn't it?

DE SAUSSURE:

It seems to me that Piaget distinguished between, on the one hand, a static situation and, on the other hand, a dynamic situation. He said that for him the solution seemed to be the dynamic solution, but in fact what we observe clinically is that there are people who adhere to the static situation and cannot get rid of it. For example, I think that the girl who pushed the chair in against the piano was not conscious of what this meant and probably she would have to become conscious of what it meant if she were to change her whole behaviour towards her mother. As long as she is not conscious of its significance she will repeat these actions or similar actions because she does not know why she does them.

PIAGET:

Of course, there can be a clinging to the past in some situations, but what I wonder is whether the past situation is always a fact and not sometimes the result of an interpretation. In the case of the girl and her piano stool, we have a piece of symbolic behaviour which of course recalls precise previous situations. It remains to be seen whether this symbolic behaviour is the result of a reaction to something which has been preserved in the unconscious, which is always there, and which is interpreted in this way, or whether it is the present representation of a present conflict which itself prolongs previous conflicts without their being exactly the same. In the case of the girl, I should not like to pass judgement; it is Mr. Erikson who should enlighten us here; but in the case of the young man he described, the clinical case which he developed at some length, without being able to deny absolutely that there is con-servation of a previous conflict I think that a large part of the second interpretation is possible.

I do not think that there are bare facts in the affective field any more than elsewhere. A fact can always lend itself to an interpretation and I think that precisely in this field the interpretation plays a fairly big role.

DE SAUSSURE:

But there are patients that we observe during long periods who always repeat the same thing, and once we manage to put a finger on the tender spot we see that they stop repeating it.

157

ZAZZO:

In the examples given by Dr. de Saussure, isn't there a stress on the pathological? Is there not some danger in starting from a pathological method in order to make up a theory of affective evolution? Perhaps we should leave out of consideration the pathological cases as explanations of affective evolution.

DE SAUSSURE:

It is exceedingly rare that anyone completes his affective development without there being more or less deep fixations and without there being more or less strong attachments at certain stages of the affective development. But actually, I am not pretending that there are necessarily fixations or stoppages. I am simply noting that in a very large number of cases stoppages do occur and particularly at certain difficult stages.

ERIKSON:

In discussing identity diffusion or any other developmental crisis we really discuss a period of life when past and future meet, when patterns of the past have to be translated into possibilities for the future. Different people under different conditions find better or worse solutions for these tasks. Obviously, then, what Professor Piaget calls 'static', remains a hindrance to change, while what he calls 'dynamic', are patterns which (as Dr. Huxley said) can adapt to new situations. I would say that patients are by definition people who ask for help in overcoming 'static' fixations, and in making 'dynamic' patterns more adaptive.

As for people who can solve this kind of matter for themselves, what you said, Professor Piaget, reminded me of a volume of letters Freud wrote at a critical period in his life to a friend in Berlin. As a young man Freud had passed through a stage in which he was intensely interested in the German philosophic movement of Nature Philosophy. He had loved Goethe's Ode to Nature and had become a physician because he wanted to 'unveil nature's secrets'. Then something happened to him, as it happens to many young people: and he concentrated all his passion on the strictest methods of the physicalistic physiology of his day, doing brain sections, and publishing papers on neurophysiology and on paralyses in children. Then relatively late he settled down as a practising neurologist. At that time he went through a severe crisis which is reflected in the letters. Attached to these letters is a very strange document, namely, something he called a 'Psychology for Neurologists', which I must say is very hard for me to understand, but which I think Grey Walter would be interested in because it describes the brain as a kind of central agency for incoming and outgoing excitation.

The letters make clear how Freud gradually applied the viewpoint and the method of brain physiology to psychology. In analogy to his work in brain physiology, where he had dissected brains at various stages of development and reconstructed the development of certain brain centres through infantile life, he made, as it were, sections at various stages of psychological development until they formed an epigenetic continuum.

I wonder if you had in mind such a transfer of a work pattern from one field to another? This sometimes throws entirely new light on the second field. But it certainly can also lead to a belated identity crisis, until the patterns prove to be transferable. For the choices which lead an individual to his identity formation include of course choices of an occupational identity and an intellectual identity, both based on the affective sources of his interests. At the same time you also have to ask what choices are possible for him in the light of his desires and inhibitions, and his special aptitudes and limitations. In addition to all this he must find recognition and through it—I don't know whether feedback is the right word here— a constant replenishment. Shaw called it a continuous 'resource'.

So I think that the identity development of a young individual is certainly not only based on the choices which he has to make because his affective sources push from behind, but also on conditions which pull him toward opportunities for accomplishment, recognition, and replenishment. But I would say that the first choices he makes, in which a full reciprocity and mutuality with the environment is established, will remain important for all his life. Anything further will be variations and applications of his original thinking.

BOWLBY:

I should like to return to Professor Piaget's alternative hypotheses which he described as the static interpretation and the dynamic interpretation of the clinical material, because I think those two alternative hypotheses underlie some, at least, of the divisions amongst psychoanalysts at the present day.

There are, I believe, many analysts who think in terms of Piaget's static interpretation and who feel that their main task is to reach back into the patient's history where the problem originated and that, once that has been reached, the problem will come unravelled and the patient 'unfixated'. The other way of looking at it—Piaget's dynamic interpretation—is that a person comes to adopt certain methods of resolving conflicts and these he persists in using through-

159

out his life. As Piaget himself put it, the person recreates the conflict and the solution in each moment of his experience in his life. Although these processes may undergo some evolution and change, some solutions seem to be such that the person is fixated in them and can't use other solutions.

These alternative ways of looking at the same phenomena lead, I think, to two different psychoanalytic techniques. There is the technique which, to give it a rather slang description, comprises 'digging up the past', burrowing for forgotten memories of past events. The alternative technique is based on observing the way in which the patient, in his relationship to the analyst, proceeds to deal with the situation in which he finds himself by using the same old maladaptive procedures. In other words one recognizes that in one's consulting room in the here and now one is presented with a first-hand demonstration of the way in which the patient has always solved his problem and which he is likely to continue in. That, of course, leads to a technique which is based on the analysis of the transference in the analytic situation.

Now, although these two techniques are not mutually exclusive—most analysts utilize both techniques in some measure—it remains true that some analysts greatly favour one end of this spectrum and other analysts greatly favour the other end. Which end they favour depends, I think, on their theoretical position. I personally favour the dynamic one, the interpretation of the here and now in the transference relationship. (See Strachey, 1934, and Rickman, 1951).

HARGREAVES:

It seems to me that there are two possible childhood reasons why you may limp. One is that in some moment of time, through some episode, you broke your calcaneus: the other is that you were born in China, and your feet were gently bound, then bound a little bit tighter, a little bit tighter still and so on. I would have thought that, in fact, both alternatives may occur, in psychological terms, in individual patients.

Some fields of therapy particularly tend to attract for treatment the kind of case for which I have used the broken calcaneus as a metaphor. That is the case in which in the middle of trying to solve one of the expected psychosocial crises of infancy and childhood the child meets some exceedingly traumatic episode, like the death of the mother that is never mentioned frankly to her. The other kind of case corresponds to the gentle binding of the feet. Lady Asquith tells in her autobiography of how every time her father passed her sitting at table, he used to straighten her shoulders and say 'Sit up,

Margot'. That is obviously as influential over ten years as a single episode, although the kind of effect is probably different. It leads not to the tendency to re-create a single traumatic episode, but to the tendency to re-create a pattern of relationships.

I think the fractures are much less common than the binding, but are inclined to be written up more because they tend to be more dramatic. I think they do, in fact, often respond to a therapy based on a static conception. The situations that arise from the binding don't get written up so frequently, or at least they didn't in the early history of psychotherapy, and often, I think, they don't respond to this type of treatment.

INHELDER:

If I understood your point of view properly, Mr. Erikson, the adult should reach a certain equilibrium or, as you call it, a feeling of 'integrity' to the extent that he is conscious of the continuity of his development. According to you, this continuity would be due to a process of 'identification'. Well, in order to get continuity and development, identification is not enough. In order that the individual at the end of his development should become something other than what he was at the beginning, a process of differentiation must also intervene. How do you envisage this process of differentiation and how would the transformation be possible if there were only identification without differentiation?

HUXLEY:

This, if I may say so, is what I was suggesting after Piaget spoke; that you have to regard attitudes, approaches and methods of solving problems as something alive, as part of the developing human organism—indeed, as organs of the organism; accordingly like everything alive they are capable in certain circumstances of developing into something different. In purely organic embryonic development, you may get an arrest of change in certain conditions. If you deprive a tadpole of its thyroid it won't metamorphose into a frog; but if you then give it the proper dose of thyroxin it resumes its interrupted development. The frog also illustrates a frequent paradox of development—the co-ordination of continuity with discontinuity. The development of the tadpole into a frog is a single continuous process; but it passes through the crisis of metamorphosis, which makes a true discontinuity between aquatic and sub-aerial existence. This idea that mental structures and complexes and so forth are alive, parts of a living organism, and therefore, can change and develop, is vital in what Bowlby and Piaget were saying.

LORENZ:

There is no real discontinuity and nothing is really static. Everything is a process, only sometimes the process is fast and sometimes it is slower. I always get muddled up by this conception of opposites: the opposite of static is dynamic, the opposite of structural is functional, and the opposite of continuity is discontinuity. There are no such contraries! There are all gradations between continuity and discontinuity, and even if I jump, the worst that will happen is the continuity of the jump—you can slow down a jump, you can make a slow motion picture of it, and the jump doesn't differ from the slowest motion in quality.

HUXLEY:

Perhaps instead of using the word 'discontinuous' we should say 'distinct'? Nothing in biology is ever completely discontinuous, but many things may be highly distinct or distinctive. May I amplify my previous example: the pattern of organization of a tadpole is highly distinct from that of the adult frog and the organism passes from one to the other by the process of metamorphosis, which introduces a high degree of discontinuity. At metamorphosis there is a rapid change from one relatively stable pattern to another; but I agree with Lorenz that the stability is only a relative stability, because there is always some degree of change going on. At any rate there are long relatively stable periods separated by short periods of rapid transformation of pattern; the latter are essentially processes of change and the former essentially processes of maintenance.

LORENZ:

And if we take a highly accelerated process, a crisis, in which you have to move from one attitude to another very quickly, you have to unbuild much before you build the other thing. If you do it slowly you will make the change in such a way that there are no crises. I think the main aspect that ought to concern us biologists is that whenever you have a period of very highly accelerated change you have a period of increased vulnerability and danger. That happens in the metamorphosis of the frog, and when a bird hatches out of an egg, and when a human person goes through puberty. These are the critical periods of quick changes. I think that the acceleration between two critical stages is what we ought to emphasize more than the absolute speed of the process.

HUXLEY:

Yes: the function of one type of process is transformation, and of the other is maintenance.

162

GREY WALTER:
At the first meeting of the group we discussed this very problem: the question of whether abrupt changes do or do not occur in children. It seems to me that we have defined it, in fact, as being the capital problem in the whole of this discussion. We decided that there probably were abrupt changes and, of course, this is very important in working out a theory of development of the nervous system, whether descriptive or analytical in the Freudian sense, or biological or cybernetic. The existence of what cyberneticians call step-functions, or relatively abrupt changes which, though not absolutely discontinuous, have a relatively very high rate of change, has a very powerful action on the whole theory, because the derivative of such a process, of course, is correspondingly large. We know that, in general, biological receptors are responsive to rates of change rather than steady states. So, an abrupt rate of change will be perceived in an exaggerated way. Thus the sort of effect that Ronald Hargreaves was talking about, where Lady Asquith had a repeated series of small gentle shocks, would not necessarily have had the same derivative value as a single sudden large one. In a simple system the two *might* be equivalent. But in a system that undergoes abrupt transition and responds mainly to rates of change, then a sudden event occurring during one of the transition periods would have an exaggerated, apparently anomalous effect. The whole subject I think is treated very well in Ashby's book (Ashby, 1952).

ERIKSON:
I think that 'continuity' and 'discontinuity', 'static', and 'dynamic' are terms with implications of particular controversies in each field. They short-circuit, as it were, what I want to discuss, namely, that a child grows in relativity to other beings that grow around him, who are themselves passing through various stages. Therefore, any stage he reaches will have a psychosocial connotation and it is that psychosocial connotation that may create a discontinuity. Now this fits with what Konrad Lorenz said in this sense—that such psycho-social discontinuities are specially dangerous during periods of great velocity of change, either in the organism or in the milieu.

By psychosocial connotation I mean something like this: there are mothers (and I presume there are cultures) who, relatively speaking, favour babies. There are others who favour older children. A boy who has got used to the fact that he is the eldest and for a while the only child has to realize that it isn't just he who is the most wonderful thing in the world, but whoever at that moment is the baby of the family. From this moment on, he can gain new status in the family only by relinquishing the rewards of being a baby and trying as quickly as possible to gain the rewards of being a big boy; one who doesn't cry, and who doesn't demand. This he may learn sooner or later, with fewer or more regressive episodes in which he tries to be a baby again. If, during such a crisis, somebody dies, or gets sick, a war breaks out, or the family moves, such changes in the various departments of life have a cumulative effect: they get too much. I, therefore, referred to the development of identity as one in which one can establish continuity out of discontinuity, or, in Huxley's words, maintenance in change. Somebody who really grows up has to maintain a ratio of components: the baby is still in him when he becomes a big boy.

LORENZ:
The difficulty is the crisis. If you are a crab you must moult in order to grow, but you must take good care to preserve the continuity of your life in the meantime, because you are very easily eaten in the process. The point that I want to bring out with this is the vulnerable state.

ERIKSON:
As for young Lady Asquith, what her father may have done all her life became humiliating for her at a particular period in her life, when it became significant in a crisis.

ZAZZO:
Certainly we should take into consideration that it is society which accentuates the stage of development and imposes on the child breaks in continuity: the beginning of the primary school is a very clear example of social discontinuity which corresponds to a new stage of psychobiological evolution. It would, therefore, be worth while comparing different situations in order to understand the formation of identity and psychological differentiation—different situations, different groups where the child is found. A little while ago you spoke about twins: this is an excellent example of the group where the individual experiences considerable difficulty in differentiating himself and where he manages with the utmost difficulty to affirm his identity. There is actually an affective and intellectual pathology of twins which shows to what extent this integration into a biological group makes identity, the affirmation of the person, difficult.

A second situation which is very general is the situation of the child within the family. Again this is a biologically determined group where the child occupies an absolute place or, more exactly, where he lives as an absolute: when another child is born, a brother or a sister, and when the structure is thus modified, the child may be profoundly disturbed: he no longer knows exactly what is his place in the group. Then to consider the school, where the child is admitted between six and seven years. Professor Wallon, establishing a connexion between his own research and that of Professor Piaget, made the following remarks about this period: on the intellectual plane the child begins to be able to understand the idea of unity on the arithmetic plane. He begins to acquire invariants, to use Piaget's expression. Simultaneously, on the social and affective plane he begins to understand himself as a unity among other unities, interchangeable unities, and it is a very important new development in the feeling of identity: he has a stronger identity because he feels himself living as one among others. It is no longer a biological group, it is a group which has a much more mobile structure and where the individuals, all of more or less the same age, can change their role, change their place and change their situation. Identity of self and differentiation are created interdependently. Here we see a discontinuity which is explainable by the psychophysiological maturation itself, where quantitative changes, which are very rapid at this age, lead to a whole restructuring of the mentality. There are also, and I would stress this, social structures which society imposes on the child—particularly the school, which involves a new reorganization.

INHELDER:

In the present discussion we seem to be imagining that everything happens as if, throughout all the mutations due to the outside environment, the child maintains his identity. Could we not envisage another hypothesis: that the child does not only go through transformations under the effect of outside factors but he also contributes actively to his own metamorphosis?

ERIKSON:

I can only say yes. The present is the elaboration (through interaction with the environment) of the child's past.

INHELDER:

He contributes to his own differentiation, to become another being different from the one he was before.

165

ERIKSON:

Let me say it this way: Identity is not the same as identification. In fact, it is exactly that which overcomes identification as a dominant mechanism. I believe that in my own field this is an important point to emphasize, namely, that the final identity of the individual is not the sum of his previous identifications but is a more highly differentiated complex in which earlier identifications become part of a more unified whole. William James once spoke of 'the self he murdered', by which he meant, I think, that particular potential person that would be the sum of all the previous identifications with which the individual cannot do anything under given conditions. William James also says how sometimes a young person wonders whether the self he killed was not the better one.

I would emphasize in this connexion that identifications in childhood are, by definition, identifications with part aspects of people and not with whole people. A child who identifies with his father cannot possibly identify with the whole father: he identifies with his size, his occupation, his potency, or with any number of these, but it is always a part aspect. Out of mere identifications a whole identity could never grow.

Now there is another aspect to this. In a functioning social system I would think a child, as he grows through the various stages of his childhood toward adolescence, is faced with a comprehensible hierarchy within his own family, a hierarchy of roles beginning with the younger siblings and ending with the grandfather, or great-grandfather, or whoever belongs to the wider family. All through childhood, this gives him some kind of a set of expectations as to what he is going to be when he grows older, and I have a feeling that already very small children can identify with a number of people in a number of respects, and establish inside a kind of hierarchy of expectation, which then must be 'verified' later on. That is why cultural change can be one of the changes that can be so traumatic for identity formation, because they break up the inner consistency of that hierarchy. This, for example, one can see clearly in Pittsburgh, where whole European villages were transferred to an industrial neighbourhood, and tried to maintain their collective—that is national and religious—identity.

What has been described in psychoanalysis as identification is, in later childhood, already pathological identification—it is what I would rather call over-identification. It implies the necessity of settling accounts with a particular person, let us say the mother or the father. I am sure every child has to do this when he is young, and every child has to do it over again at critical periods, but on the whole,

166

in a functioning family life, the child has much greater freedom in identification than our case histories would make us believe.

As to what Dr. Bowlby said, I do not want to evade the point about different psychotherapeutic philosophies in psychoanalysis, although we are apt to confuse the scientific interpretation of life data with the therapeutic interpretations given to the patient. One could answer this by referring to different periods in the development of the psychoanalytic method itself; one could answer it by referring to the various approaches to patients of different ages; and then again one could refer to patients of different syndromes, the changing epidemiology in the neuroses of our time. I would say it is best to be guided by the patient in any given situation. The kind of patient I mentioned this morning is a young person in an acute identity crisis. One will find out soon enough that he would not stand for any exclusive discussion of his past. The simple result of doing that would be that he would break down further. For one of the aspects of this whole syndrome which I will discuss later is time diffusion. In young people with identity problems the attitude towards time as such is very pathological. They feel that there is no future, and that the past is malignant. They may feel in a tremendous hurry to catch the bit of future there is or they may suffer from a slowing up of time experience, and move as if in molasses. It takes hours to wake up, it also takes hours to go to sleep, and it is very hard to adhere to any schedule at all.

Now, to take such patients and to say 'Lie on a couch and I will sit behind you, a mere screen for your free associations' is, of course, completely out of the question. Such patients come to you to find the remnant of an identity, with a last hope of a 'recognition'. You are a teacher, a master, or whatever—and not just a transferee of the old father. In fact, as I may have an opportunity to illustrate, these patients 'transfer' the very earliest experiences of selfness and otherness. But they experience these with traumatic immediacy. They want to see that you are there, and will not disintegrate or evade.

If one is called upon to help a man who has found his identity but suffers from inhibitions or anxieties that are left over from the past, the situation is different. As I said yesterday, there are, of course, neurotic inhibitions or symptoms which go together with a perfectly good identity formation. In this case, one only wants to establish that these inhibitions and phobias are the result of left-overs from the past; here an additional education, or an additional identity formation is not called for.

167

	1	2	3	4	5	6	7	8
I. INFANCY	Trust *v.* Mistrust				Unipolarity *v.* Premature Self-Differentiation			
II. EARLY CHILD-HOOD		Autonomy *v.* Shame, Doubt			Bipolarity *v.* Autism			
III. PLAY AGE			Initiative *v.* Guilt		Play-Identification *v.* (Oedipal) Phantasy Identities			
IV. SCHOOL AGE				Industry *v.* Inferiority	Work-Identification *v.* Identity Foreclosure			
V. ADOLESCENCE	Time Perspective *v.* Time Diffusion	Self-Certainty *v.* Identity Consciousness	Role-Experimentation *v.* Negative Identity	Anticipation of Achievement *v.* Work-Paralysis	Identity *v.* Identity Diffusion	Sexual Identity *v.* Bi-sexual Diffusion	Leadership Polarization *v.* Authority Diffusion	Ideological Polarization *v.* Diffusion of Ideals
VI. YOUNG ADULT					Solidarity *v.* Social Isolation	Intimacy *v.* Isolation		
VII. ADULT-HOOD							Generativity *v.* Self-Absorption	
VIII. MATURE AGE								Integrity *v.* Disgust, Despair

The Psychosocial Development of Children

ERIKSON:

I indicated yesterday just what kind of material we clinicians deal with and today I would like to indicate into what kind of orders our observations may fall. On the chart (Chart I, on opposite page) the Roman numbers mean progression in age and the Arabic ones progressive potentialities for differentiation. For the moment please pay attention to the diagonal only. The steps of the diagonal contain *the gradual unfolding of the human personality through psychosocial crises*. These crises are, of course, determined both by what, at a given time, is ready in a child to develop and what, at the same time, is prepared for him in his social system in the form of provocation, prohibition, elaboration, connotation, and so on. In the sequence given in the diagonal, you have in each box two psychosocial criteria, one a more positive, one a more negative one. The crisis consists of the conflict between these two tendencies and if the crisis is lived through positively, productively, creatively, then the 'good' criterion will outweigh the 'bad' one. This does not mean that ever in human life the 'bad' one is entirely 'overcome', nor that the accentuation of the negative one could not appear again in certain crises. There are other considerations, too, of a philosophic kind, which must keep us from treating the 'bad' criteria as preventable or something that can (or should) be prevented or cured away.

Now, if I may briefly state what is in each box. The chart makes each box equally big; this is an artefact of systematization. In any individual, or in any given culture, the ratio between the contents of the boxes can vary tremendously, but of course, only within certain systematic limits, as we pointed out when we spoke of sexual differences. As to the sequence, however, I would be rather adamant that it must not vary. The terms *basic trust* and *basic mistrust* sum-

169

marize much that has been emphasized recently in psychiatry and in public health, especially by Doctor Bowlby. He and Dr. Spitz have emphasized the circumstances which hit the specific vulnerabilities of this stage and cause lasting 'basic mistrust'. As to the *psychosocial modalities* which I wish to introduce here, the social modality of the first stage would be (in basic English which is what I started with and hope to end up with) to learn 'to get what is given' and to experience particular givers and forms of giving. Then, also in basic English, you could say that at this time the child learns 'to get somebody to give' and then, by way of a most primitive psychosocial mechanism, the child learns 'to get to be the giver'. I am sure that all languages have certain very simple designations of the basic modalities in human relationships. The first problem would be to relate the infant's means of receiving with the mother's ways of giving, and also, of course, her ways of withholding. These herald in the first crisis which comes to a head (unless otherwise accelerated) through such physiological changes as teething, which is a disturbance in the main organ of receiving, or through the second great 'cause' of this crisis—conflicts in and with the person who is the principal giver.

Of particular importance here are those states of impotent rage which are provoked in the infant when communication is jammed and he feels the victim of inner tensions that he cannot manage because the environment does not know how to alleviate them. This would be the ontogenetic source of the sense of evil, a 'basic mistrust' which combines a sense of mistrustfulness and of untrustworthiness. Here is the ontogenetic experience of the sin through which paradise was forfeited for ever. It is obviously difficult to know what mechanisms are at work at a time which is one of relative lack of differentiation between outer and inner experience, between body and mother. But this seems to be the stage to which our sickest candidates for identity diffusion regress—as Bowlby pointed out yesterday, when he rightly interpreted their dreams of the faceless parent as also connoting the fear that the patient may destroy the therapist, his new protector, as well. There seems to be an affinity between this earliest crisis of trust in the maternal environment and the adolescent crisis which concludes childhood and tests one's capacity to trust society at large: a complete and relatively unpredictable breakthrough often occurs in late adolescence.

Now at each stage I should very briefly mention its relationship to one of the major social institutions. For I wish to claim in all earnestness that certain universal and basic social institutions correspond to the stages of the life cycles and more, that they exist for and because of these life crises. For example, the crisis of trust and mistrust persists in and endangers every individual throughout life. But every individual can find it collectively annotated and, as it were, stylized in one universal institution: religion. In every prayer, in every turning toward the supernatural or superhuman there is an attempt at re-establishing the sense of trustworthiness in relation to a god, to fate, or to history. In the first stage, the infant receives, through the maternal persons, whatever 'faith in the species' is present in them. He learns to expect that people and institutions will know how to give and restore faith. More modestly, the psycho-social gain of this period can be said to be an enduring pattern for the solution of the recurring crisis between trust and mistrust. This, in homogeneous cultures, prepares the child for the collective ways of reinforcing the solution through periodical rituals.

The transition from one stage to the next accentuates one of those normative discontinuities we talked about yesterday: in order to learn to be independent the child must have learned that he can depend. I speak now of II.2 in the diagram. But let me briefly refer to I. 2, the precursor of autonomy during the trust stage. It is one of the main aspects of systematizing in an epigenetic way, that every-thing which appears in the diagonal is in some form already present in the first horizontal. Progress is a differentiation at various stages of something that has been prepared in all previous stages. Anybody who has watched babies can already see autonomy in them, a wish at times to be left alone or to be free of things which at other times they want very much. This wish occurs at that age only off and on. If it becomes too predominant too early, a factor is created which influences the ratio between trust and autonomy, and between mis-trust and doubt, and remains in some way systematically influential for the development of the further stages.

In connexion with the establishment of the sense of autonomy, let me make a few points which are really significant for all stages. Different cultures emphasize autonomy in entirely different ways, but always in ways systematically related to the rest of the culture. There is always a minimum sense of autonomy which the life style of a particular culture must insist on, and a maximum which it can tolerate. Amongst the Sioux Indians the babies all have their feet swaddled as tightly as possible; on the other hand, amongst the Yurok in California the feet are deliberately kept free so that the grandmother can massage them every day: there you have one of those differences in accentuation which (as I have tried to show in *Childhood and Society*) imply a systematic relationship not only to

171

other items of child training, but also to world-image, economy, sexual differences, etc. Then, of course, different children are entirely different in their temperamental characteristics: only in the interplay of cultural and individual style can you get what in a given individual would be a true sense of autonomy.

There is one other systematic point which I should have mentioned earlier. When I speak of stages, I refer primarily to what *results* out of a stage at the *end* of the stage. In child development a stage is often determined by what the child is *beginning* to master. I am talking about a stage as the time at the end of which the ego will master a particular conflict in such a way that the individual, as it were, can forget about it. The relative but enduring solution has become a part of him. It is like the difference between making the first steps, i.e., learning to walk—and being able to walk in such a way that one can forget the fact that one can walk and only think of where one wants to walk.

Finally, I must emphasize again, that all these stages are intrinsically related to the psychoanalytic theory of the basic drives and of the ego: unfortunately, the mere presentation of the stages will preclude a detailed discussion of this inter-relationship. The first stage was related to what, in psychoanalytic psychosexual terms, is called orality and sensory-tactile erotism. The stage of autonomy versus the stage of shame and doubt is related to anality and to muscular development. For 'libido-development' as well as 'child development' and social accentuation have in common certain modalities, such as holding on and letting go, retaining and releasing. The sphincters, as part of the muscle system, can become the dramatic place where holding on and letting go is particularly emphasized to a degree dependent on how much the culture wants to emphasize it, and how much emphasis the individual can tolerate. From intense experiences of being held on to, of holding in, of holding on, of being freed, of letting go in relation to persons, objects, and feelings, can come a sense of autonomy; that is a sense that the child can master himself and his environment *more* than he needs to be mastered and to have things done for him. This basic ratio can later influence many modalities, characterizing, in turn, basic social attitudes such as a hostile ejecting, letting loose, or repudiating, or a tolerant letting pass, letting live, letting go. The whole stage is, of course, what the Germans call 'Trotzalter'.

LORENZ:

How would you translate 'Trotz'? Spite, cussedness? Stubbornness?

172

ERIKSON:

Trutz, an earlier form of Trotz, is something more positive than mere cussedness. It rhymes with Schutz.

INHELDER:

Opposition?

LORENZ:

Entêtement? The French verb 'bouder' is a mild sort of translation. . . . in der Ecke ist . . . Trotz.

ERIKSON:

Aber wie kommt das Kind in die Ecke?

HUXLEY:

'Stubborn' is better than 'obstinate'. 'Obstinate' is more passive, 'Stubborn' implies a positive reaction.

ERIKSON:

This is a good example of how such modalities can be related to vices and virtues alike. When 'Trotz' leads to 'Trutz', you have a warrior who won't let anybody pass. When you say 'obstinate', then you have something entirely different.

MEAD:

Well, maybe you have moral courage. When we want to describe New Englanders in America, for instance, in a way that would be acceptable to New Englanders, or to people who live outside New England, you have the choice of saying they are stubborn, or they have great rock-like integrity!

ERIKSON:

So this whole stage is one in which the child learns to control himself in accordance with certain regulations demanded in the culture. If the regulations are transmitted in such a way that the child receives a good impression of the self-control of those who are delegated to control him, he should end up with a sense that all in all, given regulations and rationales, one is able to regulate oneself more than being regulated. Otherwise a deep sense of shame over being so weak and uncontrolled in comparison with other people, and a sense of doubt either in his own mechanisms of self-regulation or in the methods of regulation and self-regulation in his regulators will

173

arise. This, of course, remains a life-long problem, reflected in our laws and liberties. Their first battleground is the autonomy stage.

HUXLEY:

Up to what age do you think that stage would continue?

ERIKSON:

I should think it includes all of early childhood. In contrast to the things you might learn to *complete* in school later, the child is here primarily preoccupied with the question—who does it, and to whom is it done, am I doing it myself, or is somebody doing it to me or for me—that is the power and extent of one's *willing* something. All of this is related to sitting up, to standing up, to being able to control first a sedentary kingdom, and then a perambulatory one. Psychosocially speaking, shame has something to do with the fact that the individual who sits up and stands up has space all around him; he can suddenly be seen and judged from all sides. An increased awareness and sensitivity to the environment goes with this. In many societies this is exploited by intense shaming—laughing when the child falls down, and so on, all of which causes a very particular rage in the child, a mixture of the rage of shame, and shame over rage. This is why shame has, at least in the English language, such connotations as that one wants to sink into the ground, which means one does not stick out in space, or one wants to hide one's face, because one may not be able yet to manage the expression on one's face. I would think that blushing has a lot to do with it. I would be interested to know when children begin to blush.

LORENZ:

And then one 'loses face.'

FREMONT-SMITH:

Would you call that paranoid?

ERIKSON:

Yes, exactly. It is the origin of lifelong paranoid trends such as are present in everybody. I could relate each stage to extreme psychopathology. Paranoia itself is the extreme accentuation of obsessive doubt of what one has 'left behind', suspicious doubt of what people would do to you behind your back.

RÉMOND:

What would be the age at which children would first show shame?

174

ERIKSON:
I would like to have you discuss this question.

RÉMOND:
Personally I had the impression that this period of 'doubt' and particularly feelings of shame came later, probably after three years.

MEAD:
I should think the shame-response could appear at about nine months, but the most likely age would be around two years.

LORENZ:
I myself recall early shame, which was the shame combined with soiling. All children in our family including myself were perfectly clean at nine months. The most shameful thing that can happen to an adult is this, and after all it is no sin, it is nothing to be ashamed of. You may be ill and not at all responsible really but still, if it happens to you, it's worse than murder. There is a sense of guilt which is absolutely awful—I couldn't find an example of such an absolutely shattering sense of shame—and this is definitely acquired at less than twelve months.

ERIKSON:
In this sense shame has something to do with the feeling that one lost self-control under 'everybody's' eyes.

LORENZ:
Yes, of course, and if you find people under extreme circumstances, undernourished and so on, who start to soil themselves, it is a sign that they will die very soon because they have completely lost control of themselves.

ERIKSON:
This is very important because in children there is a corresponding experience of absolute despair.

HUXLEY:
Could you tell us approximately when children start blushing? `

ERIKSON:
I do not know.

175

GREY WALTER:

There have been studies of blushing and change of skin resistance and acceleration of the pulse and so forth as signs of autonomic responsiveness, and it is surprising how late these autonomic displays arise, at least in English children. It is probably not before four or five.

ERIKSON:

I would emphasize here again the systematic point that probably blushing appears when the child has already learned to internalize a particular type of rage which is a response to being ridiculed or looked at.

FREMONT-SMITH:

I think internalization is crucial in the whole business of conflict and I suspect that until a certain age inhibition is not possible because the cortex isn't developed sufficiently. I believe that the exaggerated autonomic responses which are the basis of psychosomatic syndromes are present only when there is an inhibition of cortical control.

ZAZZO:

I remember a discussion we had during the previous meeting where we came to compare one of my sons with one of Grey Walter's tortoises. I had stated that my son at the age of fifteen or sixteen months, as far as I remember, had a disorientation reaction in front of the mirror, with flushing and turning away from the mirror. This corresponds moreover to one important stage of development. Up to then he had not recognized himself in the mirror. Blushing, then, appeared in connexion with a recognition of an image of self, with a sudden realization.

ERIKSON:

Skirting the question of later internalization, I would say that psychosocially speaking blushing as a primitive reaction contains an affective turning against oneself and at the same time as against others.

Now the next stage I call the play age. Psychoanalytically, we would speak here of the phallic-ambulatory stage, and I would like to emphasize again that each stage is related to a pair of organ systems, one of the pair being an orifical, the other a peripheral-contact system: in stage one it was the oral area and the sensory surface, in stage two, eliminative organs and the musculature. It is here that psychosocial and psychosexual development overlap. If

176

in psychoanalysis we call this the phallic stage it is because interest in the genitals would at this time be aroused by sensations in the sexual organs, by a general awareness which is intensified by cultural ways of counterpointing the sexes at that age, and maybe, by the experiences of shame. Psychosocially speaking the main emphasis is now on motion toward goals, many of which for the child have to be play and fantasy goals. The emphasis is on initiative in the sense that the child is passionately preoccupied in reality and in fantasy with what he wants to get at, where he wants to go, what he wants to see and touch, what question he wants to understand. The selection of goals and the persistence in approaching these goals vastly outdoes the child's actual ability to gain access and to master these goals. Many of them are transferred into the area of play. Then either the goals themselves become playful goals or else toys represent the child, and the question is where can the toy automobile go.

Children at this stage take things apart, even though they can't put them together. They gradually leave the mother's house and are taken along to be shown how to fish or shoot a small bow and arrow. In primitive societies such play has a much more direct connexion with the technology than in our lives, where play has often lost its connexion with the technological world. Yet, even here you can still see the preoccupation with what are considered the outstanding tools and roles. In any given family or culture the child here has to learn somehow who may take the initiative and when and towards whom; who has access to the tools with which you get at things. He will be at this time intensely aware of the hierarchy of ages in children. Jealousy of the younger children and rivalry with the older ones is very strong. He cannot use the helpless approach of the younger ones and he cannot as yet master the approaches of the older ones. I would think this is the most common source of impotent rage at this time.

There is a great expansion and intensification of fantasy at this time, and also a great development of guilt over fantasies in which one 'approached' people or goals which belong to others, or 'approached' them in ways strictly reserved for others. This, of course, is an important aspect of what in psychoanalysis is called the Oedipus complex. One cannot return to the mother as a baby, so one now wants to, as we would say, in American at least, 'make' her in some way as a woman, or, in the case of girls, be like her and 'make' father. The same is true for the boy's relationship to the father, whose executive organs and tools, capacities and roles he does not even approach at that time and with whom already he wishes to identify. In fantasy the boy does all kinds of things as the father does them, or as he fantasies the father does them. This then becomes the soil for sinister and hidden guilt feelings, guilt feelings which must balance a secretly wild sense of unlimited initiative. This has eminently to do with the superego development, which was discussed here at a previous meeting. This guilt is already something much more internalized than shame and doubt were at the beginning, before they were linked with guilt. But I think the differences both in different cultures and in individuals are great, and my psychoanalytic colleagues will agree that for a long time we have called too many things guilt which are pre-guilt.

FREMONT-SMITH:

Could you say that there is a progressive internalization with development?

ERIKSON:

Yes. If I were talking about the development of the ego, I would use those terms, but I am talking about psychosocial development on a rather phenomenological level. The psychopathology corresponding to this stage, in general, is based on hysterical mechanisms of denial or repression. One denies goals. One represses impressions, effects, and drives. Later, paralysis may disarm an organ as an organ of aggression or reaching out, or the individual may otherwise restrict his awareness, initiative, or techniques. There are, again, both extreme pathological forms of this and those which are very close to the norm and appear as collective self-delimitations. Probably certain psychosomatic diseases which would express a greater degree of internalization of self-restriction belong here. What also belongs here is regression. Everybody who has grown up with children knows it is at this time that you have violent shifts from victorious progression to meek or demanding regression, for example, when the child becomes sick and wants to be very much a baby again. But there is also an over-compensatory exhibitionism, where a shaky initiative expresses itself in being a he-man, in self-advertising, but always with an underlying sense that one is not quite as one advertises oneself to be.

INTERVAL

ERIKSON:

Huxley reminded me of William Blake in the intermission and of Blake's saying 'The child's toys and the old man's reasons are the

178

fruit of the two seasons'. We are now at the end of the first season. The positive outcome of this play age would be that the child has enough initiative left from his disappointments and from his guilt feelings that he vigorously enters the school age and the learning of actual techniques leading to his people's technology. This next stage I call the stage of industry, or of workmanship. It is the stage at which the child forgets most of his earlier experiences, 'forgets about' much of his relationship to his family and what he wants from them, can turn to tools, objects and work situations; he can learn with others to do competitive tasks and the tasks of finishing things. The difference between initiative and workmanship would be that, in the period of initiative, the emphasis is on the goal, but very little actually gets finished. So now the child begins to manage the smaller steps which in his particular technology lead to observation in work situations. In literate society that begins with learning to write and read; in other societies it might mean being taken along by selected teachers into fishing situations or hunting situations. I think there are certain aspects of this stage which are world-wide also; though some societies would handle it in ways almost unrecognizable as similar to our own, still there are selected adults who are gifted as teachers and who are more or less chosen and entitled to take a group of children together, and show them certain important initial steps in the management of technology. In our world, literacy has to be learned first, which poses particular problems because you enter a separate school world, while of course in many societies the school is not separated from the rest. In the eastern Jewish settlements there is probably the most extreme accentuation on literacy taking you from home and mother. In certain American Indian societies there is extreme accentuation as between the mother's house and the bath house of the men. In most cultures at this time a differentiation of masculine and feminine takes place, in that these measures are primarily for the boy. There is a marked pulling away from the home, away from the mother, and towards the tools and the techniques of the particular culture. Now, some children are not quite ready for this. For any number of reasons they want to go back home as if there was something they have forgotten there. They daydream; or a guilt feeling over something they have not settled at home may keep them from enjoying the tool situation and from becoming absorbed in work completion. This, then, is the period during which the sense of inferiority (see chart) can become strongest, in that the mastery of both the preceding and the present stage has been missed. This, very often and in fact mostly, has nothing to do with the child's actual capacities or with his real intelligence, but

179

is rather a sense that as a whole person somehow one does not deserve to do, to achieve, and to succeed. As was first pointed out by Freud, this can go back to a very marked sense of sexual inferiority in comparison with the man or men at home. But then early school failure throws the child back to the guilt-problems of the initiative stage.

In psychoanalysis this is the particular period called 'latency', meaning a relative latency of psychosexual drive. In following here the psychosocial line I must consider what Freud called libido development almost as subsidiary, while if I would speak of psychosexual development I would have to consider psychosocial development subsidiary. This is a matter of the point of departure in any particular discussion. But I do feel that both points of departure are relevant and that the originally purely biological ideas of Freud have to be restated in psychosocial terms—humanized as it were—because it seems obvious that what he described as a latency and delay of genitality is to some extent the utilization by psychosocial development of certain quantities of libidinal energy.

We have already discussed the matter of *identity* (see chart). I may just add here that in identity development, what one has learned to do well counts very much. When one approaches the identity crisis one is already somebody who does such and such things well, and one is already one whom other children have called such and such a person, maybe even by a nickname or two. At the same time, secret mistrust, shame, and guilt have set into a negative inner image. In other words, a differentiation has taken place already. Secondly, the length and intensity of the identity crisis depends to a very large extent on the technological circumstances into which one is growing. In societies with a primitive technology people have a much shorter way to the full development of the sense that they know who they are within their culture. By the same token in more complicated cultures, it may be easier psychologically for certain unskilled classes, because they remain closer to the technological pursuits which a twelve-year-old and a thirteen-year-old can already manage.

Depending then on the degree of civilization, identity development in certain specialties and in people who because of inner complications can only survive in the specialties, is tremendously prolonged, maybe all the way up to twenty-five or more. What I call the school-age here, therefore, includes everything that you learn in a preparatory way, all kinds of apprenticeships and psychosocial moratoria of other kinds—graduate studies, and after-graduate studies. Some people prolong this (Veblen, for example, after college went home for seven years, just to read by himself) and the age-range is, therefore, almost impossible to state.

I think I have indicated that the identity development itself is sub-divided into a number of part-identities, such as sexual identity (what kind of a man, what kind of a woman one is), age identity (younger adolescent and older adolescent), and occupational identity: these divisions can grow at different rates, and this also depends on individual patterns as well as cultural ones. As for the sexual moratorium, it can consist of early promiscuity without personal commitment, or of a long-drawn-out period of abstinence. I think my psychoanalytic colleagues would agree that in our field we have emphasized too exclusively the mechanical consequences of either abstinence or promiscuity for the individual, and have underestimated the role and status factor in sexual behaviour. In some classes, and in some cultures, early promiscuity is so much the rule that the child has to act it out whether he is otherwise particularly motivated or not, just as in another culture or class, abstinence would be the rule. The demands can vary from sexual licence with a total lack of personal commitment, to a deep personal commitment without sexual liberties. The individual's motivations must be evaluated within such patterns.

While the vicissitudes of genital drives must be accounted for under all these conditions, we cannot simply assume that what young people 'really' want is to have intercourse. Very often what young people want from one another—though it is obviously hard to say what a person 'really' wants—is mutual delineation. The young man becomes more differentiated as a man if he mirrors himself in a girl who, at the same time, through him tries to become more of a girl, and in this sense a polarization takes place which is a necessity whatever the sexual mores.

I would especially emphasize that psychiatric ideology has done at least as much harm as it has done good by suggesting to young people who were in the process of such mutual delineation that maybe intercourse or early marriage would be the thing that would solve it all. The fact is that only two people who have learned already to delineate themselves in relation to the other sex are psychologically ready for genital mutuality. Thus sexual activity as such is not the royal road to maturity.

Identity diffusion is the item from which I took my departure yesterday morning. In horizontal V, in the chart (page 168) you will find those elements of identity diffusion which we discussed yesterday. But let me point out another principle represented by this kind of epigenetic chart. It is apparent that V.1, *time-perspective*,

181

is really a late development of what in I.1 is called *basic trust*. In other words, if young people are inclined to believe that time and history are benevolent, that there is a whole lifetime before them, space to go somewhere, and historical tradition: this would be basic trust in the form of a more differentiated time perspective. Time is not going to crush you, and time is not going to be more than you know what to do with.

MEAD:

Time is on your side.

ERIKSON:

Time is on your side, and history is on your side. It is for this reason that ideology is important for this particular age. By ideology I merely mean a coherent system of images and ideas which, among other things, gives the young person at this stage a sense that history is on his side. *Self-certainty*, V.2, would be a later development of the sense of *autonomy* (II.2). It means that now one is not only an autonomous person, one is also a person with a particular social identity. In this way, each item of the chart is related horizontally and vertically to an item that developed earlier and to an item that is developing now. So that self-certainty is determined both by the earlier development of autonomy (vertical) and by the over-all identity development (horizontal).

But here the chart should be three-dimensional, with a social dimension providing depth. For the young individual is unable to have self-certainty of his own. He must join a subculture, a movement, an organization, a clique, or a circle of the like-minded. That is why at this time fraternities, secret societies, delinquent gangs, and ideological movements give young people a sense of self-certainty which we as clinicians know they would not have reached alone.

Role experimentation (V.3) is another part aspect. Young people, depending on where they live, will try out a number of gangs, or cliques, or organizations, or movements. It is very hard for their parents to understand what makes them change from, say, a pacifist to an extreme militarist organization. The necessity to totalize one's outlook and one's associations at any given time is an adolescent trend.

Then in V.4—we have the *anticipation of achievement*. It means that whatever is one's apprenticeship one must be promised a mastership. One over-identifies with the people who teach particular achievements, and while one has to learn still to be a student and still to be an apprentice, one already learns 'wie er sich räuspert und wie er spuckt'. Then we come to V.5, i.e., *identity*, and V.6, *sexual identity*. Adolescence is at an end when one's sexual maturation is completed, *and* one's psychosexual role defined and accepted. I do not think VI.7, *leadership polarization* needs to be explained further, but it should be said that this is a further development of conscience formation. In any culture, the young person has to learn to be a leader of some and a follower of others. I call it a polarization, because these two roles are systematically related in any human society. That is why I get annoyed when questionnaires in America ask you about a particular child—'Is he a leader?' I always want to ask what kind of a follower is he, because that one has to learn also, and nobody can be a leader who has not learned to be a follower.

LORENZ:
Unless he is a megalomaniac?

ERIKSON:
That alone would not make him a leader. At the same time, I don't think anybody can be a follower who could not at any given time take over the command, at least in a small unit.

FREMONT-SMITH:
Even Hitler was a follower at one stage.

ERIKSON:
The only friend that Hitler had between the ages of sixteen and twenty has written a description of Hitler in those years, and if you want to have a ludicrous example for everything that I have been saying about adolescence you will have to read it. Hitler went through a very prolonged psychosocial moratorium during which for four years he had only this one friend, and then for two years not a single friend anywhere who could remember ever having seen him. In those four years he went around rebuilding Linz, in Austria, in his imagination. This friend not only describes him, but has sketches in his possession that Hitler gave him. He lived in Linz at that time, and as he went around rebuilding it, his friend wondered whether the more important thing for him was to tear down the houses or to rebuild them. At any rate, Hitler called this his work. He hungered, he abstained from the pleasures of life, and he abstained from friendship, and rebuilt Linz. This friend who is a very naïve—but I think, if I am a psychologist at all, a trustworthy—individual was a musician, and he felt that Hitler needed a public,

183

and he was his public. Then even that much public was too much for Hitler. He suddenly disappeared, and apparently he lived in homes for itinerant workers. When the friend later met Hitler again, Hitler was the 'Fuehrer' of the German nation which included Austria, and he had started to rebuild Linz exactly according to the plans he had drawn up as a young boy of eighteen. Indeed, one of the last things Hitler did in his bunker and in the days preceding his suicide, was to complete his plans for the opera house in Linz. Leadership polarization for a man like Hitler meant from the beginning only to be an absolute leader.

LORENZ:
You know that one can produce leadership in fish? There is chronically a strong followership. If you cut off a minnow's forebrain the fish can still eat and see, but the schooling reactions are somehow destroyed. Paradoxically, this fish becomes automatically the leader, just because it moves without any regard if someone follows him or not.

GREY WALTER:
We had a whole collection of our models at one time and several of them would go round and round the room in procession. We found that one was always in front; it would lead the procession round the room and keep them together. The one that was in front was always one that was faulty—he couldn't see. That one couldn't see the others, but they saw him and followed him. It was a very impressive demonstration of a delinquent appearing an ideal leader.

ERIKSON:
I have always felt that psychosocially speaking these two things come out of the same matrix.

LORENZ:
That just shows how perfectly fitting your expression of leadership polarization is.

ERIKSON:
Now as to *ideological polarization*—V.8. By polarization, I mean that the ideal ideological position should be sufficiently separated from the undesirable position. Here it is important to understand that identity development at its height presupposes the repudiation of otherness, at least for a period. We must understand that a young person may need something at one time which he can relinquish at

another. Prejudice of some kind cannot be ruled out by decree or by pious wishes. If ideological evil is not clearly defined in accord with the prevalent identity young people will turn against all kinds of things. Some of them are innocent enough. In one area of California at one time the left back hip pocket of boys had to be torn, and anybody who had not torn his hip pocket—well, what could one expect from a guy like that?

HUXLEY:
At Eton it was obligatory for all the boys to leave the lowest button of the waistcoat undone.

ERIKSON:
Little items like this can become the expression of distinction and repudiation, and this has a lot to do with the development of snobbishness.

HARGREAVES:
In Fighter Command during the war, the fighter pilots distinguished themselves from bomber pilots by leaving the top button of their jacket undone.

BUCKLE:
Where do you fit in the phase of change from feeling that one is a child to feeling that one is an adult, and the expectation often given by the adults for some kind of initiation into their group?

ERIKSON:
I know a few fraternity rites in America where the individual has to go through a harrowing experience for a few days, in many ways quite analogous to primitive puberty rites: he has to starve, is kept from sleeping, and gradually is scared into a kind of twilight state in which almost anything seems possible, in which he really begins to have the feeling (as the student describes it) that something is going to come to an end or a new beginning is going to be made. Such organizations share this with large ideological movements which also emphasize that one kind of world is coming to an end, and a millennium of another kind is going to start. But the important thing is that through some experience of this sort, the individual comes to feel that he is wanted, that he is reborn into a particular ideological brotherhood which is from then on more important

185

than his family. The victimization by ritual has the peculiar consequence that he feels that he has actively adopted the new way of life with all his will.

BUCKLE:

I was thinking not of the sense of ideological or sexual identity, but the way in our culture in which a child grows up by learning to do the things that men do, which operate very strongly in a purely homosexual channel; for instance drinking patterns and drinking habits. This is not a work role, it is not a sex role in the sense of sexual differentiation; it seems to be another system.

ERIKSON:

Now as to the next item, *intimacy* (VI.6): besides sexual intimacy, I think what is important here is intimacy with one's own drives and excitations as well as with the body of other people. Transitory masturbation in adolescence may thus be a step not only towards identity but also toward a sense of intimacy in the sense that the individual becomes able and willing at one time or another to face the quantities of his sexual excitement. The next step is to fuse it with the sexual excitement of others. This sexual intimacy in the psychosocial sense obviously depends on one's identity, in that only two people who are pretty sure of their own identity, can bear completely to fuse genitally with another person, and this because of the climactic nature of genitality and the loss of consciousness in the climax. All this seems tremendously dangerous to young people who have not found their identity. That is why they may be either crushed by sexual experiences, avoid them altogether, or sometimes try, as it were, to crash through to genitality, without real success.

LORENZ:

May I add this point—I am not so sure that intimacy, I mean to say, non-sexual intimacy, always comes so comparatively late in life. I think that very often character traits determining identity may develop quite early. A great percentage of my friends are people with whom I got intimate at the age of nine or ten.

ERIKSON:

With regard to young friends, that is an early selection, which must be verified and made final in late adolescence. But in some individuals and in some cultures, all of this may start much earlier.

186

LORENZ:
It has, I feel, very much to do with identity. If two boys develop a real friendship as early as that each must remain very identical with himself if they are to keep up their friendship. Indeed, the earlier-made friends give you the highest reassurance of your own identity if they endure. The highest reassurance your own identity can have is that if you meet a friend again after thirty years, you find him identical.

ERIKSON:
Yes, indeed.

HUXLEY:
May I interrupt for one moment: couldn't you have in addition to the types of intimacy you have mentioned, what might be called team intimacy or companionship intimacy, which may be very important?

ERIKSON:
Team-intimacy belongs here most definitely. Even intimate enmities and rivalries.

Now comes a word which I always apologize for—*generativity* (VII.7), which I merely use because I do not want to use the word creativity, and I don't want to use the word productivity. This designates anything you generate—your own children, the whole next generation, goods, objects or ideas. I would say again that in psychoanalysis we have omitted this further development of the libido because of our preoccupation with neurotics who could not even become 'genital' because of their infantile psychosexuality. We have, I think, understated this further development, such as the love for what one generates, which is an independent matter, not just something like—well, to mention an extreme—a transfer of anality to the organs of conception. *Self-absorption* (VII.7) doesn't have to be explained, I think, as the opposite of generativity. People who do not develop generativity of one kind or another treat themselves as children. They go on spoiling themselves, being hypochondriacally concerned with themselves, building up their whole lives as if they were their own children to be taken care of.

HUXLEY:
The pathological side of it would be narcissism.

ERIKSON:
Yes, it is a regression to narcissism. Now we come to *integrity*,

the final step, a difficult thing to discuss, and I am sure Huxley could find a quotation from William Blake which would say what I can only indicate poorly. It means really something beyond generativity, something beyond intimacy, and most of all something beyond identity. This I want to emphasize particularly, because you may come to the conclusion that I would consider the definition of one's identity the final step in life. Maybe the simplest way for me to indicate integrity would be to refer back to that very nice short phrase of Shaw's, when he looked at his own identity formation, called himself 'an actor on the stage of life', and said 'This I learned only too well'. There is something in the ageing person because of which he has to recognize the relativity of his own identity, as against that of all others, and yet has to accept his own life cycle as the only life cycle that he will ever have. For the ageing person this is not an easy thing to accept, but maybe you will agree that it is the perfection of maturity, which is supported by a universal social institution, here wisdom.

MEAD:

His own life cycle as the only *remembered* life cycle he will ever have, because half the human race feels that there is another life cycle with continuity.

ERIKSON:

Yes. You might say the individual accepts his own remembered life cycle as the point from which he looks at the great variety of other life cycles known to him, being able to encompass their relativities, and this is one aspect of wisdom.

* * *

GREY WALTER:

While Erik was speaking and describing his chart, I was trying to see whether one could translate his terms into the terms in which I try to think about this problem of maturation. This is in terms of a rather probabilistic approach to animal—or human—experience. I jotted down a set of headings, which correspond to Erik's I to VIII, and I should like to see what impression it would make on Erik in particular and on my psychiatric colleagues. I suppose, to make sense, it ought to give one an idea of what to look for in children— we see an enormous number of children, some suffering from exactly the sort of disturbances Erik has outlined, some of them normal controls. Our difficulty at the moment is to know just what observations are worth making, let alone what experiments to plan.

The scheme that Erik has suggested has brought to life some notions of my own which before have appeared quite lifeless.

The first stage that Erik outlined for us involved the question of giving and getting, getting to give and getting to be given—the trust-mistrust stage. It seems to me that from the neurophysiological standpoint, the answer which a nervous system, if it were a computer, would give back in reply to the environment at this stage, would be 'insufficient information'. That is, I am considering that in the baby-world situation the environment is questioning the nervous system: the observer or the environment is testing the baby, and the baby-computer is giving back the answer, 'not enough data' which is, of course, the answer one should get when there is not enough information supplied.

You would expect that in a recently born nervous system there would be an insufficient number of complete circuits to handle anything but the simplest situations. The simplest situation for the baby is this question of getting and giving, getting food and comfort in small quantities at regular intervals and giving signs of distress and satisfaction. Now this seems to me to produce just that state of mind, if you like, or state of brain, that one can understand by the 'trust/mistrust' contrast. Let us now reverse our point of view and think of the situation from the standpoint of the baby-computer trying to solve problems for which there are insufficient data or for which he can't handle the mass of data. It is difficult to force a computer to give an answer for which it hasn't got enough data, but you can do this for certain types of machine—you can turn a knob which makes the system less and less accurate and more and more 'trusting'. It can be persuaded to give you an approximate answer, to guess. If you ask it 'What are two and two?' it doesn't really know the answer but it can be forced to admit that it can't be more than five or less than three—it will give an approximate answer to a precise proposition. This is what one would expect to happen in a statistical theory of learning in a nervous system that was not primed with information and had not had time to collect the required data.

FREMONT-SMITH:
It was not only not primed, but it was also insufficiently developed.

GREY WALTER:
That's true, of course: if we take an anatomical analogy, for example, if we associate walking with the anatomical size of a child's legs—you still won't get him to walk before the age of, say, eight

189

months, and it won't matter what you do, the white matter just isn't there in the nervous system, whatever the size of the legs may be.

In stage II, where the antonyms are 'autonomy' against 'shame and doubt', that seems to me to be the equivalent of the use of tentative statistical criteria derived from stage I. In other words, the computer is, all the time, building up a stock of statistical criteria from experience but at this stage it can't really act on them with any confidence. It has got beyond the stage of pure trust or guesswork and has accumulated enough data to make a tentative calculation. In the simple model of learning which I presented at our last meeting—and which I maintain is the simplest possible one—there is also a stage at which data have accumulated but cannot readily be used. There is a store of information but this store is, in any useful mechano-physiologic sense 'unconscious'. It certainly has no overt effect in normal circumstances and is quite hard to detect in the machinery, but it is there, and it has the effect of giving the mechanism some degree of autonomy and of freedom of action in an emergency, because there is sufficient information for it to make trial essays of behaviour. This corresponds in stage II to the question of holding on or letting go: it is in the nature of a set of hypotheses being built up.

Here I should like to ask a question to which the answer would be very important to my theory: do you recognize an important difference, at stage II, between behaviour patterns which are based on or grow out of appetitive activity, as compared with those that grow out of defensive activities? The reason that this is important to my theory is that a purely appetitive activity, which is built up as a result of experience in the newly hatched or born creature of this type, is very easily extinguished: it has the clear characteristics of the simple Pavlovian conditioned reflex, being liable to extinction by the withholding of a reward or by the lapse of time, and it may leave no trace at all. In other words, a situation of conflict between autonomy and shame that is developed from the irregular satisfaction of an appetite, could be relatively harmless, and it could die away without treatment or insight. On the other hand, one based on irregular punishment, the exploitation of a defensive process, could be permanently dangerous, and give more sensational effects— perhaps long-term compulsive, obsessive, even paranoid states. This is according to my theory—which is a very rough one.

LORENZ:

Didn't Howard Liddell show that he could create obsessions with only negative stimuli?

GREY WALTER:

Yes, I believe that at the last meeting that was agreed to by Howard Liddell, and I think that in the case of animals there is support for it, but the situation as regards human beings is not so clear. It is not obvious to the human that defence is not an inhibition. There are all sorts of paradoxes that might arise in the human being which would make hay of this rather simple explanation, which is crucial to my particular theory.

BOWLBY:

In the psycho-analytical literature the view has frequently been expressed that fixation could be due either to over-indulgence or to frustration. I confess that I have never seen a patient in whom I thought that fixation was due to over-indulgence, and I don't share that particular view. So I agree with you.

ERIKSON:

Prohibition after over-indulgence certainly may be fixating.

GREY WALTER:

Yes, it's complicated, of course, in the human being in that sort of way. I imagine that if you let a baby over-indulge and then punish it later, something might happen which would complicate the issue. Cyberneticists have discussed the situation in which a correcting system says in effect: 'You have gone too far—go further'. There might be simple cases in which it might be effective, perhaps— the Road of Excess leading to the Palace of Wisdom.

Another question that is running through my mind all the time as I look at diagonal squares in the chart concerns the abruptness of change between these phases in the individual. Statistically, in a population, of course, you wouldn't expect a very abrupt transition, but in individuals a very rapid transition should, on the whole, have survival-value in an organism with a prolonged childhood. If there is, in fact, a fairly abrupt transition from stage to stage, in an individual, then he is less vulnerable, because the time taken to change over is shorter. This again comes out in the study of Ashby (1952), or in any cybernetic approach to the problem of maturation; if a step-function exists, then during the time when it is just about to change, to switch over (like a thermostat that's heating up and is just about to turn the heater off) it's very vulnerable—a bit of vibration and it will just go over or just go back again. What is very interesting psychiatrically is that during this period of change-over, when the contact, so to say, is just wobbling between phase I and phase II, or phase II and phase III, it can easily get into an unstable vacillating state, with anticipation and regression back again. In other words, the effect of some catastrophe in the child's life, in one of its short vulnerable periods of change-over might well be mainly a regression to an earlier stage. It might even go right down through the sequence again, like Snakes and Ladders.

HARGREAVES:
The speeding up of the phase of transition reduces the period of vulnerability but makes it more dangerous while it lasts, doesn't it?

GREY WALTER:
It reduces the number of casualties, but increases the risk of serious injury in those to whom something unlucky happens. This, as Ronald Hargreaves implies, should produce in the population a very skew distribution of neurotics; instead of having a normal distribution of neurosis (like the distribution of stature or weight) in which most people are slightly neurotic, a few are very neurotic, and a few are not neurotic at all, you get most of the population untraumatized, but the minority very heavily traumatized. These are the ones that are unlucky enough to get hit when they are running from one trench to the other, so to speak. Study of the population statistics of neurosis might throw some light on the very important problem of whether or not there are abrupt changes in the neurophysiological and psychological behaviour of children. If one compared the distribution of the various types of neurosis, one might get some idea whether some types were due to conflicts experienced during the vulnerable change-over phases.

If you have a number of smooth changes that follow an S-shaped curve, each rising slowly but influencing each other, it is easy to show that the effect of the combination is to produce an abrupt step-function. If you have a very large number of fairly slow changes, all working together, the effect is to produce a sudden change. Fessard (1954) illustrated this very nicely in the Proceedings of the Laurentian Symposium on Brain Mechanisms and Consciousness. One doesn't have to suppose that anything terribly romantic happens, like millions of neurones suddenly being myelinated at the same time, but simply a few processes of gradual change connected in series would produce, in fact, a very abrupt change in behaviour, with all the possibilities for vacillation and regression, which would be diagnostic of this process. Of course, from the point of view of the theory of learning, that would be extremely important, because it means that the system would change its law, that as you go from

192

square to square in Erik's schema, in between the two would be a vacillation of law.

This is very difficult to put in words but it is clearly defined in Ashby's book (1952) where there are diagrams, showing what is meant by an ultra-stable system, in which the representative point in the system may run off the edge of its stable platform and can then find another platform, another system of operation, and quite new laws. You cannot have a smooth transition from one to the other, because the two together may be totally unstable. This again might be a point in child behaviour; if a child is, for some constitutional reason, or as a result of an illness or accident, trying to make too smooth a transition from one stage to the other and finds himself operating under two laws at once, life may be quite confusing and, as Ashby shows again, such a state may produce very dramatic, violent vacillation or oscillation of the whole mechanism.

The third stage, shown on the chart as 'initiative' as against 'guilt', represents in my terms the stage when a creature is acting on hypotheses which have now been built up during the first two stages, but which have still to be confirmed by test. I suggest that the initiative phase in development, assuming that it is a healthy one, is a stage where there is quite a bundle of home-made hypotheses in the brain, which are still to be tested, and this is the testing time of these hypotheses. In other words, the brain computer has extracted from experience a contingency rating high enough to permit action, but it is not yet a 'natural law', it is only a notion, a limited theory. The baby computer, or now the child computer, in the play age, is testing out the hypotheses which it has built up, still, most of them, not at all conscious—or not in any useful sense conscious. It is playing with these ideas and making experiments which, later on, if we go down column 3, become role-experimentation, the rehearsal stage. The rehearsal stage is really a development of the essential activity, of play. Play as a whole is a test of initiative combined with rule-keeping, even in sub-primate species. What we call 'make-believe' is synonymous with 'als ob' reasoning.

I think the rate of change gets less abrupt here: and this is what intrigues me in this whole system: if there is an advantage in rapid transition, if there is a survival value in terms of a diminished probability of being hurt, then why is it that mankind has done so well with such a long period of infancy? It would seem possible that one of the compensatory factors is the existence of step-changes within this long period of development. Although there is a long period of immaturity, at each stage the system is fairly stable, so that the person climbs to maturity, not up a long slope but in a series

193

N

of fairly abrupt steps, and the advantage for anyone standing on a step is that within its limits it is level, whereas if you are standing on a ramp it is all sloping.

That seems a possibility, because in the next stage, stage IV, where we have the industry and inferiority contrast, there an entirely new thing is happening, which interests me very much in relation to learning theory, the organism at this stage is having to accept *predigested statistics* at school. This is the school age and he is dealing with preselected contingency computations, with the 'facts of life', the facts of the three Rs, history and geography; it seems to me the acceptance or non-acceptance of this is exactly what is important in the school age; consistent failure on the part of the organism in its earlier phases to work out the later parts of the statistical sum will mean that it will be unable to accept the predigested material at a later stage. It can only either accept or reject, it has no way of making a tentative judgement. In the case of human children a schoolchild who has not acquired his statistical criteria in play or whose brain has not developed normally is still forced by the culture to go to school or to accept instruction or initiation which it can either accept or reject. It cannot make a tentative judgement; so you may get a child who is in love with school and authority, accepts everything he is told, is completely taken in by any sort of doctrine or myth and in the extreme is the fanatical member of a party. On the other hand, the same situation may result in a child who is completely, profoundly, sceptical, rejects every attempt to instruct or teach him, irrespective of so-called intelligence, and becomes the pariah, the outcast, the cynic who will not accept anything and who later on refuses to accept any ideology or general notion at all, and becomes the desperate nihilist. In case this approach should seem really too naïve, remember that at this stage I must postulate that the child has accumulated a colossal number of hypotheses about the world and it is this gorgeous network of ideas of inter-relationships between things and events that seems to me to enfold the idea of self, to be weaving the identity. On this web I suggest there is imprinted the identity of the individual who has gone through these experiences. At this stage approaching adolescence, one can imagine that the system will begin to extract general laws. A complicated model would do the same thing, but it would have to be quite an elaborate one. This seems to me then to be the stage of abstraction and the formulation of some 'laws of nature'.

The notion of causality will arise here too; and the connexion between experience and notions of causality seems to me to be of paramount importance in understanding young people. We regulate our lives very much on notions of causality, and at some stage of his development every sane individual has to build up and accept for himself or take over from somebody else an elaborate system of causal relationships. But this can only be achieved if the foundations have been laid in the earlier stages. Of course, as a corollary of the development from a statistical to a causal world, in the model or the child one would see the elaboration of *dei ex machina*—gods outside the machine—of common causes and first causes and so forth. This too is an effect that one might observe quite easily with a very simple set of models; one would begin to find the machine giving out little chits like you get from a weighing machine—it would be easy for the machine to issue apt little aphorisms about the world in general, because if it were forced to give a short answer to a really complicated problem, it could only give an aphoristic answer. This stage is then the age of aphorism too, when the child is beginning to quote proverbs and carry around little tags, and put mottoes up on its wall, feeling they must contain secrets of the universe.

Another characteristic of this phase would be constant testing by excess. This seems to be an interesting point about, perhaps, most animals. Certainly mammals show this constantly going to extremes in everything, of testing ideas to breaking point. This is sometimes called the scientific method, but it's really the method of the adolescent who goes through a score of crazes before settling down. If you want to know how a toy works, you can go on fiddling with it until it breaks—and any scientific hypothesis has to be tested to destruction, or should be testable to destruction.

It is only up to stage V that I have developed this notion from the point of view of statistical neurophysiology. From that stage the brain is full, so to speak, and after that what happens is determined more by the fullness and effectiveness of the brain pattern, and the interaction with cultural influences. This is just an essay in the transposition of these notions of development to the general theory of learning by association. There may well be objective physiological correlates of these stages which one can measure and record and contrast and, as a matter of fact, this is what I propose to try to do; to use this sort of schema to grade the children we see and try to construct some correlative objective table, bearing in mind that we tend to see more psychopathological than normal material. This may really be very helpful, because pathology takes processes to extremes, and you can see these conditions almost in a pure culture sometimes. This schema of Erik's is about the first realistic diagram that we have seen that tells us anything about the psychobiological development of the child.

BUCKLE:
Perhaps Grey could continue the account into what would happen to people when they got a little older; some psychological data suggest that the brain begins to deteriorate in certain ways from thirty or forty years onwards. What would be the analogy to that in your models?

GREY WALTER:
Well, that's rather difficult to say for certain because even the simple models have a large number of possibilities—a great many things might happen in the way of wearing out or deteriorating. There is one effect, though, that I should expect to find regularly if the model I am considering would include reflexive processes, instinctive or IRM ones and associative ones as well—something like a combination of the three models Olga, Irma and Cora I demonstrated at our meeting last year. This compound model contains several series of relay elements leading to one another and would exaggerate the effect of any *general* process such as illness or ageing. Consequently, a slight change in general conditions must have a dramatic effect both on the pattern of instinctive behaviour and on the criteria for the adoption of novel conditioned modifications. In the living brain, I should expect that the effect of age would be seen first and most as a specific action on any functional region or system of the brain in which there is a cascade or series of nerve elements. The diffuse projection systems in brain-stem and thalamus are such an arrangement of elaborate filters in series connexion. Any general change in metabolism which affected them would have an exaggerated effect on behaviour since it would seem that all sensory information must pass through these filters. The reason why general effects are exaggerated in these conditions was discussed at our meeting last year; briefly it is because the number of elements appears as the exponent in the equation. For example, if some general change, such as arteriosclerosis, reduces the transmission probability or the efficiency of synaptic transmission by one half, then in a series or cascade system the overall reduction is a half of a half of a half and so on. If there are ten relays the overall reduction would be by a factor of 1024. Similar effects would be seen with any neurotropic hormone or dietary change. Konrad reminded us once of the effects of artificial but apparently adequate diet on the elaborate instinctive feeding behaviour of shrikes. In humans too, dramatic mental changes occur with inanition. Helweg-Larsen *et al.* (1952) described the specific effects of starvation as: impairment of memory, reduced spontaneous cerebration, disappearance of libido, in-

196

difference. This even in a German concentration camp where there was still some chance of survival, and morale was otherwise surprisingly high. These are precisely the changes one would expect if the chain of diffuse relays were affected. So the first sign of ageing might well be to simplify instincts and to restrict the ability to learn. These effects might not always be seen as social deterioration—in the early stages, behaviour would seem more austere and discriminating—but in the extreme it would be dull and dirty. I would suggest that a sufficient explanation for these changes is the metabolic endocrinological and vascular decline which is so common from middle-age on.

FREMONT-SMITH:

There is some indication that, as the central nervous system ages, cells drop out. If we go back to your computing model, supposing you have given your model all its information, and then supposing you were to take out, in a random way, every tenth or hundredth tube, how would this affect the computing apparatus as compared to taking them out before information was fed in?

GREY WALTER:

Well, it would make very little difference in maturity until you cut it down to nearly fifty per cent.

FREMONT-SMITH:

Well, that I think corresponds to reality in a very interesting way.

HUXLEY:

I was very much interested in Erikson's chart. We may disagree with this or that detail, but we have now a comprehensive statement of the method of psychobiological development and the possibility of its continuity. It is not uniform but epigenetic, as you rightly said, in that novelty arises during the process. Novelty arises through two methods—first of all through the development of new mechanisms of change, and secondly through the effects of the environment becoming incorporated into the process. To take a parallel from biology, new mechanisms arise during the development of the sea-urchin or the frog, or indeed, almost any organism. First of all, there is the action of the genes in relation to a polarized gradient-field. Then there is the stage of mosaic determination well illustrated in vertebrate embryology, in which each part is chemically pre-determined to do something precise and specific. And then there are the mechanisms of interrelations—the endocrine system and the

197

influence of one part on another. Further, all these mechanisms operate in relation to the environment. For instance, environmental influence may distort the gradient-fields; once they are distorted beyond a certain degree then you will get permanent structural distortion. Thus in Stockard's experiments with lithium, the head of the gradient is depressed, and so you get microcephalous or cyclopic embryos.

Another interesting analogy is this: in psychological as in biological development, as Erikson stressed, the structuring which arises in each of his phases persists in some measure into the later ones. So in a sense the first stage is the most important; in psychiatry it is useful to go back to the past, though you can often detect it by looking at the present state of affairs.

That marked changes in personality structure can be imposed upon one from without, is obvious from all our experiences; for instance, there is the way in which so many of our acquaintances have had a really very different type of personality structure imposed on them by having to go to fight in the army or navy or air force. Again, many people have had a different personality structure imposed on them through sexual love—by falling madly in love, with emphasis on the word 'madly'. This brings up an earlier point, namely that in this madness of love, you often find the analogy or metaphor of surrender being used by the lover. The man or the woman feels that he is surrendering his will or his identity to somebody else, and that does mean a real personality change. Even when you get over it, something new has got incorporated in your personality structure.

Then another point: I have just been reading Bronowski's (1943) very interesting book on William Blake, in which many things seem to me to be highly relevant to what various people here have been saying, and especially, perhaps, Erikson.

For instance, Blake began one of his books with a statement that 'Without contraries is no progression. Attraction and repulsion, reason and energy, love and hate, are necessary to human existence. From these contraries spring what the religious call Good and Evil' (here we have Blake hitting on the idea of the dialectic long before Hegel expressed it in formal terms). A further aspect of this is his constant emphasis on the two opposites of Innocence and Experience. Bronowski gives a penetrating analysis of Blake's treatment of these 'two contrary states of the human soul'. 'The symbol of innocence, up to this time in Blake's career, had been the child; the symbol of experience, mazy and manifold as Blake's symbol of the hypocrite, and as fascinating, is the father.' The innocent child has to grow up and experience what it means to be a father, but he can only do so by killing something, either within or outside himself.

This passage too is extremely illuminating, where he speaks of the way in which, somehow, man has got to combine innocence and experience: 'Although the life of the senses is one-sided, it is part of the whole life, innocence and experience together; and only by way of this life can we enter a whole life. The tree is the knowledge of good and evil. The child is freed from the tree only when these are become one. For he is freed by murder.' The deepest meaning of the particular poem which he is analysing is, he writes, 'that innocence becomes experience by energy; and to that end must submit to becoming guilty, because it must work in the flesh.' I think this is very illuminating because it makes nonsense of many statements about sin. For instance, that you can get rid of evil and pain by denying their existence, like the Christian Scientists; or the conclusion implicit in my brother's book *Grey Eminence* (Huxley, 1941) that Père Joseph was always animated by the best motives, but because he had to put them into action they always went wrong; so the final moral to be drawn was that you ought never to act at all. In Blake you have a reconciliation of that dilemma. You must act if you are to live and grow, but you can't help sometimes acting wrongly; you can't help bringing in evil; you can't help causing pain, either to yourself or somebody else, but this is necessary for life and growth and the fullness of experience. Good and evil find their reconciliation in progressive development.

Also Blake brought in the psychosocial aspect. For instance, Blake often speaks about how society was imposing limitations and frustrations on man's free activities, and how it eventually becomes necessary to have some sort of a revolution, which would lead to a new type of society. Such a process could go on *ad infinitum* in a series of cycles; but, as Bronowski points out, Blake saw that beyond Society is Man. Society, up till now, has been either something which we just have to accept and which does put a brake on our activities; or else it has been exalted into a kind of super-individual, something more important than the individual man, as in certain aspects of Marxist Communism, Nazism and Fascism. But in the long run we shall find out how to make society not an end, but a means to an end, and the end will be the fulfilment of man. So, as he says somewhere, no revolution is the last: you always have to go on toward greater and further possibilities.

This interests me a great deal because it links up with what people like Simpson, and myself, and Rensch are gradually getting at in

199

modern evolution theory. Simpson (1953) points out in his latest book, *The Major Features of Evolution*, that at least ten times as many species have become extinct in the course of evolution as have survived. I would add that of those which have survived, at least ten times, perhaps one hundred times, as many have become stabilized at a certain level of organization, apparently indefinitely and inevitably, as those which have continued to advance. Only a very small minority has been able to progress to a new and higher form of organization. Even of those which have been capable of advance to a higher level of organization, most are self-limiting or self-limited. Thus all specializations inevitably, so far as we can see, come eventually to an end. You can't have a horse which is more horse-like than a modern horse: you can have a zebra and an ass, but they are all modern horses. As far as we can see there is no way of continuing that trend towards further specialization. Or you can have something which eventually introduces some limitation which was unsuspected at the beginning: the most striking example is that of insect respiration, pointed out by Krogh many years ago. Insects adopted the method of breathing by tracheae. This is more efficient than breathing by lungs, so long as you remain small. But it becomes completely inefficient when you get large, so that it is physiologically impossible to have an insect as big as a rat. As they never could grow large, they could never have large brains, they never could have a large number of brain neurones, and therefore, could never have so many possibilities of combination, and had to rely more on instinct and less on plasticity and intelligence of behaviour. And if it hadn't been for that, none of us would have been here now!

This leads on to the fact, which I think is relevant to our discussion, both from the individual and the psychosocial point of view, that in Blake's words, no revolution is the last. Every now and then in biological evolution you get a type which is capable of achieving large-scale biological improvement by evolving to a higher level of organization. Furthermore, the only satisfactory definition of biological process that I have ever been able to find is this: biological improvement or advance, which does not stand in the way of further general improvement of type. This is very much in line with Bertalanffy's (1952) ideas about open biological development, with Charles Morris' (1948) ideas about personal development, in his book, 'The Open Self', with ideas about the Open Society, and with the general idea of unlimited possibilities still open before us. This in turn brings up, I think, something very relevant to what you were saying about ideology.

In the past, most ideologies have definitely been backwardly directed, resistant to the idea of change. Our problem today is whether we can get ideologies which are either partially or wholly change-promoting. The answer is yes, of course we can. For instance, in regard to scientific method, we have long adopted the idea that change is possible and desirable, and we practise and encourage it. So far, however, this is mainly in the field of the natural sciences, though of course it is beginning in the social sciences too. Then it has been done on a larger and more extensive scale, in ideologies like Marxism, where the whole emphasis is on change: but the possibilities are still limited by the authoritarian nature of the system, and secondly by the fact that Marxism is an apocalyptic or millenary ideology, envisaging an ideal final state beyond which there can be no further progress. In both these ways it ceases to be an open system. An open social system would be, I should imagine, one which would provide the best environment for the open personality to develop.

The question arises, can you get a cultural ideology which would be an ideology of change, and which would apply to all aspects of human activity, and still be open in the sense that it does not contemplate any final state? In little groups such as ours here something of the sort can certainly be achieved. Such groups can be self-moving systems, dynamic, but reasonably stable with a self-regulating equilibrium of change towards some sort of improvement in knowledge—which, however, is unknown to their members at the time. This linking up of the assurance of possibilities to be realized with the idea that we don't know precisely what is coming, and yet trying to define it a little more, is extremely relevant. Whether you can make an ideology of this sort have as much compelling force as an ideology which claims certitude about everything, I don't know. But we ought to try.

Finally, you said that history is on our side. I agree, but would prefer to enlarge that view. We can be on the side, not merely of history but also of destiny in general, using destiny to include history in the past and possibilities in the future.

There is one other point. We discussed the matter of personality distortion imposed by society, or by social relations, or by frustration, and also the idea of supernormal stimuli in animals. It is quite clear, I think, that you can get a cultural distortion which produces a totally abnormal or subnormal result, but it is equally clear that you can have a cultural milieu which acts as a supernormal stimulus to totally new degrees of achievement. As Konrad Lorenz knows, jackdaws and ravens can count just as well as human beings, provided that the human beings don't have the use of verbal symbols.

But the possession of verbal symbols and then a long history of people using those symbols to build up mathematical systems, together with an educational system encouraging the learning of them, has led to the development of higher mathematics out of something that was originally no higher, so far as we know, than the capacities of a jackdaw. Much of Kroeber's work points in the same direction. He showed that the cultural milieu is necessary to bring out genius. A genius doesn't just happen anyhow: he is somebody who is capable of being stimulated by a particular cultural milieu to do something exceptional in it.

LORENZ:

May I just say one word. You will find a paper by a Swiss psychologist and sociologist, Jean Gebser (1954), on the ideology of the Western world, which says that our ideology is and ought to be that we don't have an ideology. You will find there very nearly exactly the same thoughts about ideologies which you have just propounded.

FREMONT-SMITH:

There is one other element which comes into the concept of an ideology which accepts, favours and encourages change, that is that it has got to accept, favour and encourage change at a progressively accelerating rate.

HUXLEY:

Well, not necessarily. Change could go too fast. You might have, and I am sure Grey Walter would agree with me, a system which promoted change at such a rate that human beings couldn't keep up with it. You have got to aim at an optimum tempo of change.

FREMONT-SMITH:

Well, isn't everything that is happening now happening at a progressively accelerating rate?

HUXLEY:

Yes, but I think there is bound to be a limit to such development sooner or later.

GREY WALTER:

I think we are reaching the limit now in the communication of information. If you discover two facts, there are three possible classes of relation between the facts, but if you discover one hundred facts, the number of possible relations becomes impossibly large. I think the evolution of scientific thinking is already slowing down.

HUXLEY:

You will find that with every major evolutionary improvement or advance you get a sudden change (or rather a relatively sudden one, for it may take millions of years) producing a new type and its radiation. Then you get the improvement of each of those types, which we call specialization; this trend goes more slowly and eventually bends over and becomes asymptotic to stability. The same thing seems to happen with human activities. For instance, it happened with ploughing by primitive methods. After a series of improvements, ploughing ceased to change in essentials: it became stabilized. Today, though, we are getting new mechanical methods, which are superseding the original type of plough.

HARGREAVES:

I think Dr. Huxley really has brought us round to the idea that Erik mentioned yesterday, when he talked about the individual having the capacity to establish his identity if the culture gives him room for it. Really, I feel that we have been talking about what kind of culture gives people room to establish an identity—but the trouble about the sciences is not only the vastness of its mass of facts, but also that to some extent scientists are all 'zoot suiters'. One characteristic of the zoot suiters or the teddy boys is that there is a lot of gang warfare between the different groups, and the shared ideology, say of biochemists, includes the idea that all psychiatrists are mad. And the shared ideology of all psychiatrists includes similar ideas about other groups, so that there isn't at present, except in comparatively few people, a wider shared ideology about the future of the human race. It seems to me another element that is important is a culture which is 'open-ended'—having a loyalty to the unknown future of the human race, which includes not only the idea of change, but the idea of heterogeneity, because homogeneous change seems to me to be no change, in that everybody has to change together, like a flock of birds that all take off at once.

HUXLEY:

That was really implicit in my remarks. When I spoke of realizing possibilities, I should have said realizing *more* possibilities, which implies greater variety. This is just what biological evolution has achieved—a richer as well as a more intensively efficient manifestation of life.

MEAD:

I think that perhaps this particular chart of Erik's raises more complications than the equivalent psychosexual chart, in that he is using words here that have been arrived at deviously and perhaps, in some instances, dubiously, as compromises out of the common stock of our information. Now in Erik's chart of pregenital psychosexual development (see Vol. IV, in press), when one uses only diagrams of zones and modes which can be handled formally, and does not have to include such words as guilt or autonomy, it is considerably easier to see the way in which these modes are grounded in stages of development of the organism. It is not awfully difficult to see why the oral stage comes before the stage that involves locomotor mechanisms, or why a stage that involves taking in receptively precedes the stage of going out and getting. But the interest of this conference has been centred on the problem of identity and the psychosocial chart includes many descriptive literary words that we should not lose sight of. But this scheme is based on a definite relationship to the structure of the organism and to the types of behaviour which show formal relationships to, say, taking in, receiving, grasping, moving towards, relinquishing, which do not have to be handled in terms of words which have philosophical connotations, such as the autonomy that comes after getting rid of guilt or the autonomy that comes before one is capable of it.

ERIKSON:
I may add that I would be more than grateful to any member of this group who wants to suggest to me that the use of a certain word is undesirable, because of its connotation either in another language or in a neighbouring field.

GREY WALTER:
There is a term that is very current in England just now in circles concerned with delinquency and that is the term 'responsibility'. There is a great deal of discussion as to whether a given criminal is responsible for his actions. A Royal Commission is considering whether a lay jury could decide whether an individual criminal could be regarded as being fully responsible, or to what degree he is responsible—in the most difficult case, for murder. I wonder whether that might be a word that could find a place on your chart—the sense of responsibility or irresponsibility is obviously associated with feelings of guilt and seems to play a large part in normal social development. There is also the general question, which is high-lighted by capital punishment, as to whether societies are responsible for their criminals. Very vague and unsatisfactory discussions are held around this, but there is a general cultural feeling of joint and universal responsibility and/or the difficulty of deciding whether a person is uniquely responsible for his actions.

We know that in fact clinically there are various degrees of responsibility, it is a state that develops slowly and isn't born in a baby. It
would be hard to say whether a child of a certain age is responsible
for any particular class of action. Do you think that there is a term
which could find a place somewhere here?

ERIKSON:
I am not sure I can answer you sufficiently. This matter of the
responsibility of the young delinquent is, of course, primarily a legal
question. Psychologically speaking, he is at a stage where he is both
still a child and already an adult and it would be hard to test how
much he is one or the other. The only contribution that my formulations would make to this is the question as to whether we, as
representatives of society, could recognize an individual who chose
delinquency or criminality as a negative identity and a perverse kind
of psychosocial moratorium, as it were. There must be more definite
criteria which differentiate between a state of identity diffusion of a
schizophrenic, a hysterical, and a delinquent type. Once we come to
understand this and can specify the criteria and find tests or find
criteria in existing tests, we should be able to establish to what
extent a young person made a choice of a negative identity.

GREY WALTER:
So many of our young delinquents, as everyone knows, don't
blame themselves for their offences. They say they are sorry they are
caught, but the recidivists have a very general character of blaming
something else. They are often told what to blame by the psychiatric
social worker! They blame their family or a broken home; they can
read now, so they know what the causes of delinquency are supposed
to be. But, apart from that, they have a fairly spontaneous sense of
irresponsibility. They haven't got any degree of autonomy, they
haven't got a feeling of personal guilt. They don't consider that
freedom of action implies responsibility for action.

ERIKSON:
I would rather speak of a miscarriage of the development of the
sense of guilt. From what we know from working with young criminals, which for me is only a very occasional occupation, I do not
think one could ever say that they really have no guilt feelings. It
belongs to the negative identity which they show to society, that
they must insist they have no guilt. I would not even say the so-called
psychopathic delinquent has no sense of guilt, but he has lost all
trust that any show of guilt would get him anywhere. I think that a

205

sense of responsibility if put on the chart would be part of the resolution of the alternative of initiative and guilt. This is related to what we call super-ego development, quite obviously, because it is the super-ego which will tell you what goals you may still go after or even fantasy about, or what intentions and acts will call forth inner signals of guilt.

GREY WALTER:

The reason I am particularly intrigued by your placing it just there is that we have plenty of evidence that the majority of recidivist juvenile delinquents, who have on the whole a *good* attitude to their mother and to their leisure occupations, their companions, their social relations, have a brain activity which would put them in a much lower age category than their chronological, endocrine, intellectual or anatomical age. Some people call this 'immaturity' or retarded development of the brain activity but I am not sure it is just immaturity. It is something a bit more subtle than that. Perhaps one should use the term suggested for other types of infantilism: ateleiosis. It looks as though there is quite a large group of young delinquents, perhaps 60 per cent. to 70 per cent. of them, who have some disturbance around about the period which you describe as the play age, in which their sense of responsibility should be developing; post or propter hoc the previous stage, which you call the doubting stage, remains the most prominent feature of their lives. They are full of doubts and vacillations. We call the result ductility, because socially these people are easily led. Any influence that comes to bear on them will direct them to crime or reform. When one influence is removed, then they will revert again to some other influence. They are recidivists because they are constantly being tempted to delinquency, and constantly being reformed. Their whole juvenile existence is a history of vacillations from one mode of behaviour to the other, even after the age of eighteen, and it seems that here we may find a close correlation between this tentative scheme which you developed by impressionistic methods, and the objective results of the measurement of brain activity. Non-criminal adults of this type seem to retain a love for episodic adventure sandwiched between periods of withdrawal and seclusion.

BOWLBY:

It seems to me that the sense of responsibility is related to self-identification: you cannot be responsible for yourself unless you know all major aspects of yourself. The characteristic thing about the psychopathic delinquent and other disturbed personalities is that

206

there are large parts of himself which he does not know. A conscious sense of guilt is dependent on a conflict both aspects of which are in some measure conscious. The psychopath keeps part of his feelings out of consciousness. Many psychopaths identify only with their greedy, hostile and cruel feelings and deny the existence in themselves of any kindly feelings. I have treated such a person myself. It was apparent to me that she was really very shamefaced towards me: she regarded me as good and she regarded herself as someone who was so unbelievably bad that there were no prospects of her ever being accepted by me—indeed, of her ever being an acceptable member of society. She managed to avoid conscious guilt by the simple expedient of claiming that her way of life was was much better than anyone else's. She was, in fact, a prostitute, a Lesbian and a thief and she did all these things in a big way claiming that she was not in the least guilty about them. The problem with her was to help her recognize her own feelings of generosity and kindness and love, all of which she had the utmost difficulty in tolerating because, of course, they came into such acute conflict with greedy and sexual aspects of herself.

And that brings me to identification. In the problems of identification which one meets in adolescents, the question is why they can't help swinging from one extreme to another—why their identifications are so incompatible. Erikson's boy wanted to be both a monk and a trumpet player and you cannot easily be both: these two identifications represent two incompatible ways of life. It seems to me that the main problem with which we are all faced in the process of growing up is that of making a tolerable and compatible synthesis out of a number of manifestly incompatible components. We hate and we love, we are greedy and we are generous, we are kind and we are cruel. These things are literally incompatible and it is only by making some tolerable synthesis out of these incompatibilities that we develop any sort of unity. The task for the individual as he grows up is not only to own to all these different parts of himself but gradually to relate them in some self-balancing unity.

The question then arises as to why some people are unable to relate and unify these different parts of themselves in a satisfactory way. I think we know of at least two main reasons why people find this difficult or impossible, and I daresay there are many others besides. One set of conditions is when the strength of these conflicting impulses is persistently above a certain threshold. If a child is deprived, his need for his mother's company may be persistently and embarrassingly high over a long period; similarly his hatred of her may also become persistently and embarrassingly high over this same period. Obviously, the higher the intensity of these impulses, the more they conflict with each other and the more difficult are they to integrate. Another common way in which an important component comes to be omitted from the developing personality is through a parent disapproving very strongly of a particular aspect of a child. If a parent regards sexuality, for instance, as being an intolerable, disagreeable thing, the child doesn't accept his sexuality and doesn't identify himself with it and thus sexuality becomes a non-integrated part of his personality. As a result he may grow up with the incompatible identifications of being a prude and a peeping-Tom. Naturally, we all develop manifold identifications. Provided they are compatible it is all right; it is the incompatible identifications based on unresolved conflicts that lead to disunity of the personality.

MEAD:

What are the conditions of disassociation in which you do or do not own to this part of your personality?

BOWLBY:

I think one could refer to the notions of forgivability and unforgivability. Provided something is forgivable one can own to it, but if it is unforgivable one cannot. It is characteristic of neurotic patients that they regard something or other in their own impulse-life as being unforgivable, unmanageable, uncontrollable, and this is why it has to be divorced from the rest of their personalities.

HUXLEY:

Isn't it a fact, John, that sex is rather peculiar among all these factors in that at puberty suddenly something happens to you, apparently from outside your ego, though actually from inside your body from the circulating sex-hormones, and a change is imposed on you?

BOWLBY:

I don't want to give the impression that I think these dissociations are entirely due to adult disapproval. That, I think, is only one source of them. The other source is that the powerfulness of the drive is so disagreeable and frightening that we are inclined to say that we don't want to have anything to do with the drive, and to disown it.

MEAD:

Unmanageable within the full framework of the society—the

child, for example, who has an enormously greater than usual greed, even though the adults might be kind, would nevertheless, feel it as much more exaggerated than its companions and other people around it.

BOWLBY:

Not only that, but the magnitude of his greed creates an even bigger conflict with his own love and concern for the object—say his mother. If both impulses are at high level, the clash which results is much more unmanageable than if they are both at more modest levels.

HUXLEY:

Dr. Bowlby started off by talking about the incompatibility between being a monk and being a trumpeter in most societies, and then went back to the incompatibility between different inner urges. This is to my mind something very different. There are two different kinds of incompatibility—the incompatibilities between your own impulses which arise automatically, and the incompatibilities between different possibilities of identity. There is a point which I wanted to bring up before and forgot—on the subject of hobbies. I think it is very important, in any complex society where there is a high degree of specialization, to provide the possibility of really satisfying hobbies. When this is not forthcoming you may get the most extraordinary phenomena, one of the most remarkable of which happened in England during this century. A rather dry, meticulous civil servant, William Sharp, invented a second personality for himself whom he called Fiona Macleod. 'She' wrote remarkable poems all full of Celtic twilight, and he actually corresponded with her—he corresponded with the other half of his dual personality. This was an extreme, almost pathological case—but many people can increase the variety of their identities, which is probably a good thing. I know a very distinguished man, I won't mention his name, who behaves and looks quite differently when he is in the Athenaeum Club from when he is in the Savile!

ERIKSON:

I would like to have seen the handwriting of the 'two' correspondents.

O

HUXLEY:
I believe it is possible to do so.

LORENZ:
Before I put a question I want to make a statement, which may be very much a matter of course, but maybe other people feel like me. Erikson's statement about negative identity suddenly makes comprehensible to me the hitherto incomprehensible fact that there are villains. You see, in my religion, there is a God but no devil—evil is just lack of the creative and not something negative trying to create in the opposite direction.

I was confronted repeatedly in my life with people who actually did the contrary of good, which we call evil, which didn't make sense at all, but now I suddenly understand that there are fixed personalities who know and feel perfectly what is 'good' but are forced, by the mechanism which you demonstrated, to do the opposite.

HUXLEY:
'Evil be thou my good!'

LORENZ:
And the other thing—I have been for a long time greatly intrigued with the question of the hysterical character that has, if I may use Grey Walter's terminology a specially high ductility of identity. It is characteristic of the hysterical character that he can identify successively with incredibly different people, and be comrades with people in speech and thought and gesture and outlook. Of course, this is not the only characteristic of the hysterical character, but it is one of the most important, and I was struggling in vain with the question, 'How does the conception of hysterical suggestibility, of hysterical lack of backbone in time, overlap and coincide with your conception of identity diffusion?' Is the hysterical character a special case of identity dispersal or diffusion, or is identity dispersal as a special phenomenon one condition for the appearance of what we call a hysterical character? The two syndromes must meet somewhere. What happens when an hysterical character gets a good and well-marked identity dispersal?

ERIKSON:
I can only take refuge in the position that there are different preconditions for identity conflicts, and one of them is an hysterical

personality. The hysterical identity conflict is different from a paranoid or other one, and the hysterical one is, indeed, characterized by what you called the ductility of identification. The hysteric has a collection of identity fragments, each of which he can display as complete at different times. Very often the hysterical character has a histrionic quality, and if everything works out nicely, that is if he lives at the right time, and finds the right profession, then he can elaborate what you call the ductility of identification into being different people at different times, let us say as actor, orator, politician, psychiatrist, etc. So what comes first? I don't know. In every such question so much depends on what kind of individual he is, and at what time of history he lives, and in what part of his society. In a primitive tribe a woman with an outstanding hysterical character may be a medicine-woman, because she is the one who can identify with conditions in other people and always can quickly guess what is wrong. To utilize such a gift, however, it is important that, in addition to the ability to identify quickly with somebody else, one must be able quickly to regain one's own identity. This is really the art of diagnosis, and of all empathy—psychological, artistic, and histrionic.

LORENZ:
Now it is characteristic of some hysterics, of these role-playing characters, that they can play the role so long as they have an audience, and not before themselves. These people are happy as long as they have an audience who believes in them, but have to change their milieus because after one audience has seen through them and does not play up to them any more they have to turn to a new milieu, which is not yet warned against the different roles of their façade. As they are out for approval they have to adapt the whole identity to each new audience and so the poor things have to change from one identity to another.

DE SAUSSURE:
Charles Odier considered that one of the criteria of maturity was what he called 'endogenous securization'—the ability to achieve for oneself a feeling of security, that is to say, a security which would come not from outside but from inside. Do you not think that this criterion of 'endogenous securization' would be a fairly important criterion in one of your diagonal squares? It seems to me that it is also closely linked to the problem of responsibility and to

211

that of identity. One can only achieve identity once one has a feeling of inner security.

ZAZZO:

According to you, what are the conditions of this endogenous securization, of this feeling of internal security? There are probably conditions which are exogenous?

DE SAUSSURE:

Of course, in order to achieve endogenous security one must have a certain exogenous security. But let us say that for a long time the child feels himself to be secure if he is in tune with his environment; but there comes a time when the child has had sufficient experience to be able to rest on this experience and to feel himself in security even if he is out of tune with his environment.

It is a process of interiorization, a process where Piaget's ideas of socialization experiences, etc. are probably very much concerned. I think this would be a fairly descriptive term for one of these stages— internal securization.

ERIKSON:

I would say that security after all can be expected during childhood and adolescence only in relation to a particularly restricted group of people. The baby will certainly feel secure only with one or two persons, especially at critical times. Each of the stages which I outlined coincides with an extension of the social radius of interaction: from the family to the known 'world'. Therefore, with each crisis, security has to be re-established within a wider radius, from a mother or maternal person to that of parental persons in general, which would include two polarized people like father and mother, to the basic family, to the neighbourhood, to the peer-group, to the apprenticeship organization and so on. Each of the early securities is basic for the later one, but it has first to find its own establishment in its own social radius, and in that sense I believe the security problem continues all the way through and is not added at any particular time.

RÉMOND:

Mr. Erikson, I have the impression that I have not heard your explanation of the succession of ideas which you have in column 5 in your table, from 'bipolarity' to 'identity'. Could you go over again what you wanted to show in this vertical column?

This column is really very tentative. But I will do the best I can. In I, 5 I have the term *unipolarity*. I mean by that the great and as yet undisturbed security of the baby in his complete dependence on the maternal environment, which will be disturbed only if he prematurely feels the loss of and thus the dependence on the mother. It looks as if this unity gave him an inner pole which does not make it necessary to differentiate himself from that original matrix. That is why I contrast premature differentiation of self, a premature sense of being separate, with a sense of unipolarity. Gradually, however, he does differentiate himself, for any number of reasons, which culminate in the sense of autonomy. During this process he has to establish with his mother what I call a *bipolarity*, because once he has lost the feeling that he is one with her, there have to be two that interplay in a way of mutuality. And his security lies in his ability to interplay with her.

I know that I should make a string of quotation marks around the word '*autism*', (see III.4) but I do believe that children who do not develop a bipolarity with their mothers and selected other people withdraw and develop a bipolarization with their own fantasy life which I call 'psychosocial autism' which some children develop for some time without ever being autistic in the psychiatric sense. In extreme cases you can observe that autistic children play with their own vision, or their own hearing. In other words, they would not use their eyes to bipolarize with an object outside, but act as if they were looking at their own vision; or they go around with fingers in their ears, and, as it were, play with their own audition. There are all number of gradations from what you might call psychosocial 'autism' to what would be a psychiatric 'autism'.

Then the third step, *play identification* (III.5) would be the kind of security a child can develop after he is able to interact intensively with a number of people. I would think that during the initiative stage great security is derived from identification in play with others, and identification with others in playing. By *Oedipal fantasy identifications*, I mean that the child would in his fantasies identify, for example, with a very dangerous or very powerful father, or a very endangered mother. This would be alleviated by the child's ability to have a rich play-life and to identify playfully with a great number of people and to measure himself and his own strength versus their strength in play. But if this fails, then we have a child who has to fight giants in his own fantasy, and there is no corrective, except an unrealistic identification with them. There is no testing of reality, and no convincing experience of the fact that most adults are rela-

213

tively benign people and do not annihilate you if you fight them playfully.

Then the next stage would be *work identification*, which probably is in itself already somewhat clearer, because it means an identification with people who know how to do certain things and to complete them. That has an enormous importance for the child's anticipated place within his technology and therefore is a more direct precursor of identity. In work identification you can see the special problem of children to whom the plumber or the gardener or the policeman are more tangible people than the father who, say, every morning, takes a brief case and goes to work, where the child has no idea what he does all day. *Identity foreclosure* would be any development, such as precocity or gifts or character development, which 'types' the child so early, that he does not develop even a normal and necessary amount of identity diffusion.

There is one aspect about the juvenile offender I want to come back to. In juvenile offenders you find a strange combination of an extreme sense of social sensitivity and of a 'lack of guilt'. In other words, the people you are talking about (whenever it was that they started to offend) regressed, I would say, in psychological terms to the state of shame, and cannot manage it. There is an interesting American ballad, of the man who is on the gallows, and is to be executed, and people mill about and want to watch the spectacle. In this ballad he repeats the refrain, 'God damn your eyes', meaning 'You cannot damn me with your eyes—God damn all of your eyes for looking at me'. Now this is, I would think, one of the basic criminal positions and often has to do with an intense shaming of the small child before the guilt stage, in which case the guilt stage never fully develops. Maybe this is one of the conflicts in the kind of person you have in mind.

HUXLEY:

Erik, you said that you find your own assurance by finding out what you mean most to others. But surely you've got to think of 'others' in a highly abstract way when you are dealing with the solitary genius—I mean a man like Spinoza, or Leonardo, who never communicated the contents of his notebooks to any actual others, or the artist who paints pictures merely to satisfy himself. I quite see that such cases can be brought into your schema, but you have got to transcend all crude or simple formulations of it.

ERIKSON:
I spoke of young people, and I don't know Spinoza's identity problems as a young person. You will find in Shaw's autobiography, that he admits to having 'always been a stranger in this world and . . . at home only with the mighty dead'. Rare people can afford to establish an identity in their historical time and then move on to a position where they may really feel solidarity only with those very few who sit on the lonely mountain tops of history basing their final identity on a common integrity. These are often people in whose late adolescence a kind of premature integrity arises, which makes them in many ways old, and yet preserves a certain child-likeness. But even the people on mountain tops maintain some kind of identity based on a sincere sense of tradition, and most of all, on the deepest solidarity with the human race.

REFERENCES

ASHBY, W. R. (1952). *Design for a brain*, London.

BERTALANFFY, L. VON (1952). *Problems of life: an evaluation of modern biological thought*, London.

BIRCH, H. (1954). In: *Josiah Macy Conference on Group Processes*, 1954, New York.

BRONOWSKI, J. (1943). *William Blake, 1757-1827; a man without a mask*, London.

ERIKSON, E. H. (1950). *Childhood and society*, New York. Swedish Edition: (1954) *Barnet och Samballet*, Stockholm; Japanese Edition: (1954) Tokyo; German Edition (in press) *Kindheit und Gesellschaft*, Zürich.

ERIKSON, E. H. (1950). Growth and Crises of the 'Healthy Personality'. In: *Symposium on the Healthy Personality*, Supplement II to the Transactions of the Fourth Conference on Problems of Infancy and Childhood, June 8-9 and July 3-4, edited by Milton J. E. Senn. (Prepared for the White House Conference, December 1950). Josiah Macy, Jr. Foundation, New York.
German Translation: (1953) *Wachstum und Krisen der gesunden Personlichkeit*, Stuttgart, also in *Psyche*, Heidelberg, 7, 1, 112.

ERIKSON, E. H. (1951). Sex differences in the play configuration of preadolescents. *Amer. J. Orthopsychiat.* **21**, 667.

ERIKSON, E. H. (in press). *The problem of identity*.

FESSARD, A. (1954). In: *Brain mechanisms and consciousness*, Oxford.

FRANCK, K. and ROSEN, E. (1949). A projective test of masculinity-feminity, *J. Consult. Psychol.* **13**, 247.

GEBSER, J. (1954). *Strukturwandel Europaischen Geistes*, Essen.

HART, C. W. M. (1955). *Contrasts between prepubertal and pubertal education*. In: *Education and anthropology*, Stanford, p. 271.

HAYES, C. (1951). *The ape in our house*, New York.

HELWEG-LARSEN, P., HOFFMEYER, H., KIELER, J., THAYSEN, E. H. THAYSEN, J. H., THYGESEN, P. and WULFF, M. H. (1952). *Famine disease in German concentration camps*, Copenhagen.

HENRY, J. (1941). *Jungle people, a Kaingàng tribe of the highlands of Brazil*, New York.

HERSEY, R. B. (1931). Emotional cycles in man. *J. ment. Sci.* **77**, 151 (reprinted in 1944 by the Foundation for the Study of Cycles, New York).

HONZIK, M. P. (1951). Sex differences in the occurrence of materials in the play constructions of preadolescents, *Child Development*, **22**, 15.

HUXLEY, A. (1941). *Grey Eminence*, London.

KESTENBERG, J. (in press), *J. Amer. psychoan. Soc.*

MANN, T. (1948). *Joseph and his brothers*, New York.

217

MEAD, M. (1935). *Sex and temperament in three primitive societies*, New York (reprinted in: *From the South Seas*, New York (1939) and as a Mentor Book, New York (1950); English edition: London (1935); Spanish edition: *Sexo y temperamento*, Buenos Aires (1947); Swedish edition: *Kvinnligt, Manligt, Mänskligt*; Stockholm (1948)).

MEAD, M. (1947). On the implications for anthropology of the Gesell-Ilg approach to maturation, *Amer. Anthropol*, **49**, 69.

MEAD, M. (1949). *Male and female*, New York (English edition: London, 1949; German edition; *Mann und Weib*, Zurich, 1955).

MEAD, M. (1955). *The implications of insight. II.* In: *Childhood in contemporary cultures*, ed. Mead, M. and Wolfenstein, M., Chicago, p. 449.

MOLL, A. (1889). *Der Hypnotismus*, Berlin.

MORGAN, L. H. (1907). *Ancient Society*, Chicago.

MORRIS, C. (1948). *The open self*, New York.

PIAGET, J. and INHELDER, B. (1948). *La Représentation de l'espace chez l'enfant*, Paris.

RICKMAN, J. (1951). Methodology and thought in psychopathology, *Brit. J. med. Psychol.* **24**, 1.

SAUSSURE, R. de (1929). *La Méthode psychanalytique*, Paris.

SAUSSURE, R. de (1939). *Le Miracle grec*, Paris.

SAUSSURE, R. de (1950). *Psychoanalysis and history.* In: *Psychoanalysis and the social sciences*, 1949; New York, vol. **2**, p. 7.

SEARS, P. S. (1953). Child-rearing factors related to playing sex-typed roles, *Amer. Psychol.* **8**, 431.

SHANNON, C. E. and WEAVER, W. (1949). *The mathematical theory of communication*, Urbana.

SIMPSON, D. G. (1953). *The major features of evolution*, New York.

STRACHEY, J. (1934). The nature of the therapeutic action of psychoanalysis, *Int. J. Psycho-Anal.* **15**, 127.

WINTERBOTTOM, J. M. (1929). Studies in sexual phenomena, *Proc. zool. Soc.*

WOLFENSTEIN, M. (1945). *The impact of a children's story on mothers and children*, Washington.

Index

219

Horses, 46
Huckleberry Finn, 58
Huxley, Aldous, 199
Huxley, Julian, biography, 14–15
Hymen, 74–5; in animals, 75
Hypnosis, 139
Hysterical character, 210–11

Iatmul, 40, 42, 54–5
Identification, 161, 207; in childhood, 166; and identity, 166; Oedipal fantasy, 213; pathological, 166; play, 166; work, 214
Identity, 183; and identification, 166; meaning of, 142; negative, 151–2, 205; sense of, 133, 142; sexual, 183
Identity consciousness, 151
Identity development, 180–1
Identity diffusion, 16, 143ff.; components of, 151ff.; example of, 144ff.
Identity foreclosure, 214
Identity formation, 142
Ideology, 182, 200–1; shared, 203
Imitation, unlearned preference for, 69
Immaturity, 206
Incompatibilities, synthesis of, 207–9
Industry, stage of, 179
Initiation ceremonies, 39, 89
Initiative: of male and female, 71–2; and workmanship, 179
Innocence, and experience, 198–9
Insects, breathing of, 200
Integrity, 187–8
Intelligence: continuity in, 155; limit of, 133
Internalization, 176
International understanding, 37
Interpretation: static and dynamic, 156ff.; women and, 61
Intimacy, 186–7; team, 187
Invention, women and, 60
Isolation, 153–4

James, William, 166
Japan, 23
Job-rehearsal, 154
Joseph, Père, 199

Kaingang, 76
Kastenberg, Judith, 73–4
Klimpfinger, Sylvia, 69
Knitting, 60
Kroeber, 202
Krogh, 200

Language: and sex, 48; symbolic play as, 118–20
Latency, 72ff., 180
Lawfulness, and noise, 121–3
Leadership polarization, 183–4
Leisure, elaboration of, 64
Leonardo da Vinci, 214
Lepchas, 76
Libido-development, 172, 180
Liddell, Howard, 190–1
Life cycle, 188
Linz, 183–4
Literacy, 179
Love: ethology of, 18; and personality change, 198
Lowenfeld, Margaret, 118

Macfarlane, Jean Walker, 91
Macleod, Fiona, 209
Males, relation to infants, 32–3
Malinowski, B., 26
Mammals, parental instinct in, 33
Mann, Thomas, 137
Manus, 40-1, 52, 68, 83, 87-8
Marriages, transvestite, 29
Marxism, 201
Masculine protest, 63
Masculinity, devaluation of, 39
Masturbation, and intimacy, 186
Mathematics, 61, 62
Matriarchy, 24ff.; as myth, 49–50
Matrilineal societies, 26
Mead, Margaret, 17
Mechanical ability, 62

221

222

For Product Safety Concerns and Information please contact our EU
representative GPSR@taylorandfrancis.com
Taylor & Francis Verlag GmbH, Kaufingerstraße 24, 80331 München, Germany

www.ingramcontent.com/pod-product-compliance
Lightning Source LLC
Chambersburg PA
CBHW070413270326
41926CB00014B/2798